Death
to
Beauty

Death
to
Beauty

The Transformative
History of Botox

EUGENE M. HELVESTON, MD

INDIANA UNIVERSITY PRESS

This book is a publication of

Indiana University Press
Office of Scholarly Publishing
Herman B Wells Library 350
1320 East 10th Street
Bloomington, Indiana 47405 USA

iupress.org

Manufactured in the United States of America

First printing 2024

Cataloging information is available from the Library of Congress.
ISBN 978-0-253-06780-7 (hardback)
ISBN 978-0-253-06782-1 (ebook)

For all my teachers who informed, inspired, and prevailed

CONTENTS

AUTHOR'S NOTE

Myriad words and hundreds of articles have already been written about Botox. My purpose with this book is not to compete, or even try. Instead, I aim to describe the unique and far-reaching accomplishments of a single man: Dr. Alan Scott. Most of the events described took place during the first thirty years of his practice as an ophthalmologist, when he took an idea and turned it into a drug approved by the FDA.

Although Scott failed to create a pharmacological treatment to replace or stand beside incisional surgery for treatment of strabismus,[1] he did develop a drug that treats millions of people for a wide range of other conditions and sells in the billions each year.

This book is about how Scott—on his own initiative, working independently, and with limited funds, assisted by a small group of colleagues and a few experts for technical help and advice—transformed the world's deadliest toxin into a human-safe drug. Much of the story is told using Scott's own words, as he helped with this book during the last six months of his life.

Readers might question, Did Alan Scott succeed or fail? The drug he created, Botox, did not have the impact he hoped for. And, although it has earned profits for many, Scott received little financial benefit.

I didn't have the chance to ask that question, but here is my take.

Alan Scott's purpose was to ask questions and find answers—which he did. He did not strive to make a lot of money and he did not. Instead, he created a blockbuster drug that alleviates suffering and promotes well-being in millions of people worldwide.

I say Alan Scott was a winner.

PREFACE

It was the summer of 2021, and the country was still in the grip of the COVID-19 shutdown. It was a time of reflection for many. One thought that struck me was the history of Botox and the amazing man who made it happen. Botox is a big deal today, and I knew that how this drug came to be safe for human use would make a great story—but if it was going to be told, I had to write it now because only a few of us who used Botox in trials were still alive to tell the story firsthand.

Botox is a cultural phenomenon. A noun, a verb, and an adjective, it is a drug that is familiar to hundreds of millions worldwide, with tens of millions using it for a range of treatments. Botox smooths facial wrinkles, controls migraine pain, straightens misaligned eyes, calms hyperactive bladders, and much more. This molecule, found in nature, generates sales in the multibillions of dollars worldwide, under several different names. Botox is the brand synonymous with this drug, as Kleenex is for facial tissues. Yet few people know that two centuries ago, this lethal toxin was a dealer of death in epidemic proportions.

In 1822, Dr. Justinus Kerner, a district health officer dealing with botulism poisoning in southern Germany, made a daring prediction: "The fatty acid [from the blood sausage] could be of benefit in many diseases." He was right.

Thanks to Dr. Alan B. Scott, today, two hundred years later, this once dreaded toxin is a drug that treats rather than creates human maladies. *Death to Beauty* describes the monumental feat of Scott, a practicing ophthalmologist in San Francisco who also worked as a part-time independent researcher without a regular source of funding. Alan Scott's work on the project began in 1961, and on December 29, 1989, his drug (at the time it was called Oculinum) received FDA approval. Incredibly, in the process, Scott spent just over four million dollars—unlike the hundreds of millions or even a billion dollars usually spent in developing a new drug today!

As an ophthalmologist of the same era, I knew Alan professionally beginning in the 1970s, followed his research, and joined the open clinical trial of botulinum toxin type A for the treatment of strabismus (misaligned eyes) and dystonia (muscle spasm) in 1982. In the 1950s, young men like us, and a few women, who studied in medical school and were graduating to internships, were unmarried or, in a few cases, just recently hitched. Starchy white uniforms, often including a shirt and a tie, were de rigueur. A hospital patient's routine laboratory admission workup was done by a student or house officer in a small lab on the ward. Biopsies and lumbar punctures were often performed at the bedside or in a nearby treatment room. For every inpatient, a detailed handwritten history and physical examination was recorded on their chart. Intensive care units had not been established, and critically ill patients, like those suffering a heart attack, were frequently attended with a nightlong vigil. Wages were low, meals were free, hours were long, and camaraderie prevailed. I recall members of our silent generation looking ahead with confidence, optimism, and a can-do spirit—and this attitude describes Alan B. Scott to a tee.

For the saga of Botox to be told from firsthand perspectives, there was no time to waste. I phoned Alan and asked if he would help me write this story. I needed to hear in his own words how he started with a deadly toxin and ended up with Botox. He answered immediately, "Sure, let's see what happens." We were in it together, and I was confident Alan would hold up his part. And he did.

We worked on the project from June 2021 through November 2021, connecting via Zoom, phone calls, email, and regular mail. Then, shortly after Thanksgiving, two upcoming Zoom sessions were rescheduled for reasons relating to Alan's health. Nine days before Christmas, I received the devastating news that Alan Scott had died on December 16, 2021—six months shy of his ninetieth birthday. I wish he could have seen this finished book that he had helped write. I am grateful he participated in the project as long as he did. Alan had answered most of my questions and the writing was nearly done. I had hoped the book would be a ninetieth birthday present for him.

—Gene Helveston, MD
Indianapolis, July 8, 2022

ACKNOWLEDGMENTS

"Sure, let's see what happens."

This straightforward, unqualified answer from Alan Scott when I asked him if he would help me tell the story of the development of Botox is the reason I went ahead with the project. From the first day, Lynda Smallwood, who has been a part of the team for thirty years, was always there doing whatever was necessary to keep things moving, including offering encouragement when needed most. Mary Jo Zazueta got the project started by encouraging me to pursue a publisher and continued to provide wise counsel, finishing with her always superb job of editing as the manuscript went to the Indiana University Press.

Ed O'Malley, a student turned teacher, provided comments that kept the "ship off the rocks" in both fact and style as he said, "I know you'll hate me but . . ." Marianne Raab read the manuscript, and her insightful comments improved the book and made me wish I had been a student in Professor Raab's classroom. Fritz Lalendorf added his newsman's style where needed.

Eric Johnson shared his extensive knowledge with botulinum toxin management in the lab with Dr. Edward Schantz at the Wisconsin Food Safety Institute during clinical trials. Daniel Drachman, who coached Alan Scott in the handling of botulinum toxin in the beginning, generously shared his experience with me and was both gracious and forthcoming. Bill Hanke, a loyal friend, contributed by sharing his own clinical experience with the toxin and offered valuable comments on the manuscript. Jean Carruthers described her special role in introducing the cosmetic/aesthetic uses of Botox. David Josephson introduced Kristi George, who explained how a neurologist in training learned about Botox, sought mentors, and now employs it in her practice daily. Jackie Lehmer generously shared insights about Scott's unflagging interest in life and medicine, shared photos, and gave me a book written by her friend Ruth Scott describing the building of the Scott family home.

Bill Good told of his experience with Alan dealing with administrative issues, and Bruce Spivey added information about Scott and the California Pacific Medical Center. Andy Pickett provided valuable information about the future of the "toxins." This book dwells on the history. Morton Goldberg read an early chapter, and his positivity was a boost. Elbert Magoon, who was a student and associate of Scott, shared generously during hours of conversation over the months.

David Guyton offered insights about his father and contributed a photo of him holding a two-year-old future Dr. Guyton, the first of ten! Owen Lehmer, introduced to me by his grandmother, described his experience with Dr. Scott in one of his last projects with strabismus. Daryel Ellis backed up and, when needed, corrected my recollections of when we were partners in practice at the beginning of the clinical trials. He also shared the chicken story.

My family provided support, each in their own way—Martha, Lisa, David, Derek, Henry, Ali, Abigail, Charlie, Caroline, and Fred. Each listened patiently when I answered their simple question with a harangue, telling them more than they may have intended to hear. Thank you all for your interest, support, and patience.

My thanks to those who served as readers: Derek Sprunger, David Plager, Margaret Simpson, Jo Lesher, Elbert Magoon, Marianne Raab, Ed O'Malley, Vince Mihalik, and Elizabeth Simpson. I gave you versions of the work that were too early and likely undeserving of the scrutiny you gave them. When this happened, you "could have taken me to the woodshed." I deserved it. You can be sure I learned something from the unique input from each.

The team at Your Good Life, who were there to keep the candle lit and kept the writing going, were Rosemary and Bruce Hume and Sandy Hamilton.

My thanks also to the many at Marquette who asked, "How's the book coming?"

Chris Brown did a stellar job with the illustrations and was patient with me when I made changes along the way. You are the consummate professional and a pleasure to work with.

My thanks to David Hulsey at Indiana University Press, who was my first contact and guardian angel, and to Dan Crissman, who was always there to answer my pressing questions. Also, thanks to Lesley Bolton and the team at IU Press.

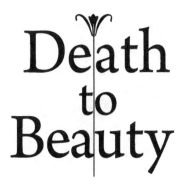

Death
to
Beauty

1

Clostridium Botulinum

The bacterium Clostridium botulinum *has been on earth for a billion years. In the last two hundred years, through the efforts of a few dedicated people, this single-cell life form and its lethal toxin have been miraculously transformed. This amazing story begins with death and culminates with a purified and diluted* Clostridium botulinum *toxin type A that was approved for human use by the Food and Drug Administration.*

Alan Brown Scott was an ordinary man who led a small team that accomplished the extraordinary feat of developing Botox. This Californian, who could be called taciturn, finished training as an ophthalmologist and elected to pursue a unique career path. He divided his time and effort equally while consolidating his focus. He treated patients in his office with the tools available to the practice of medicine *then* and worked in his laboratory searching for new methods to be used *tomorrow.*

After spending a decade studying how human extraocular muscles worked, Scott started to look for a method to change eye alignment without using surgery. Finding the right substance, he injected a potent toxin into the extraocular muscle of a monkey. The year was 1972. It worked and had a lasting effect. This was the first step in his search for a novel way to treat patients with abnormal alignment of the eyes, otherwise known as *strabismus.*

Building on these results, Scott became the first person to inject the world's most lethal poison into a human. After this, he launched the most remarkable drug development story of the century—perhaps of all time![1]

The toxin Scott employed is produced by *Clostridium botulinum.* The effect of this bacterium was noticed for the first time in the late eighteenth century, when unexplained deaths occurred in epidemic proportions in southern Germany. A study of the deaths led to blame being placed on a common food—blood sausage. The sausage contained a fatty material that was thought to contain a toxic substance. This discovery was a start, but much more work was needed to isolate the pure toxin embedded in the fat—the kind of meticulous work carried out by scientists in a laboratory, peeling away until the pure molecule of toxin is exposed and can be dealt with for what it is.[2]

Two characters in this story played pivotal roles, one at the beginning and the other at the end. In the century and a half between them were many others who toiled to uncover the mysteries of this toxin, speaking only to it and to the disease it caused. In their special roles, however, these two men *introduced* the toxin to patients and explained what it could do for them. The men were Justinus Kerner and Alan Scott.

In 1822, Kerner identified a toxin-laden fatty substance that caused a fatal disease in his patients. When he put a dab of the fat on his tongue and felt a sensation in his throat, he predicted the toxin could treat a hyper-excited nervous system in a human. In 1978, Alan Scott fulfilled Kerner's prophecy when he became the first person to inject botulinum toxin into the eye muscle of a human to weaken the effect of that muscle. Each man was speaking to a human audience on behalf of the toxin, which could be likened to a ventriloquist's dummy on their knee. Kerner and Scott provided the voice and took responsibility for the message that the toxin delivered. The scientists of the intervening years who worked to purify the toxin and explain its mechanism perfected the substance that would define the dummy on Scott's knee (purified toxin) and to which Scott would finally give voice.

The narrator in the story—me—can be likened to an interested bystander pulling the curtains when the show starts. I remain in the wings as an observer, looking on and participating in a small way. I was a reviewer of Scott's initial grant proposal to the National Institutes of Health (NIH) at the beginning of the seventies. He described clearly the project employing botulinum toxin, and it was exciting. I championed it during the review process. I was just one. Others on the panel must have agreed. This grant, the only one I know of that Scott received from the NIH, was approved. That grant was only the beginning of the story of Alan Scott and his relationship with botulinum toxin. This association with *Clostridium botulinum* and its toxin defined Scott's life's work. His devotion to the project that resulted in the approval of botulinum toxin as a drug began immediately after he completed training and continued with no letup for more than sixty years.

The earliest records that suggest a link between sickness and death from botulism poisoning appear in the edict of Emperor Leo VI of Byzantium (886–912), which restricted the manufacture of blood sausage (although the edict might have been issued to comply with religious beliefs that forbade ingesting blood, "a wicked invention due to the gluttony of mankind").[3] Other evidence linking blood sausage and poisoning was a tasteless powder extracted from the sausage and dried in anaerobic conditions. This powder had been suggested by shamans to Indian maharajas as a method to poison enemies.[4]

A well-documented early outbreak of botulism poisoning associated with blood sausage occurred in 1793 in the southwest German village of Bad Wildbad. In this outbreak, thirteen people were affected and six died. Several more outbreaks occurred in the area over the next twenty years, and the causes were initially elusive. Because a dilated pupil was a common finding, atropine poisoning was suspected but later discarded. Also, hydrocyanic acid or prussic acid was blamed. This also was discarded in favor of a biological toxin as the cause. Professor Johann Heinrich Ferdinand von Autenrieth, a physician and respected authority at the University of Tübingen, suspected blood sausage was producing the biological poison. This pointed researchers in what proved to be the right direction.

A breakdown in society caused hardship for the population during the Napoleonic Wars (1803–1815) and resulted in poor sanitation and food shortages. Blood sausage was made with raw meat, vegetables, spices, and blood stuffed inside casings of animal intestine and became a food staple. During preparation, these sausages were routinely allowed to stand at room temperature—an environment that proved to be favorable for unchecked growth of bacteria. Autenrieth further blamed "housewives for the poisoning by saying they did not dunk the sausages long enough in boiling water." They pulled the sausages out too soon because they wanted to "prevent [them] from bursting"—the authorities were right.[5]

A comprehensive, scientifically based study of the illness and death caused by ingesting tainted blood sausage was launched around 1817 by Justinus Kerner (1786–1862). Kerner was a young district health officer who displayed the genius and persistence that was a common trait in those who worked at uncovering the secrets of botulinum toxin. Kerner started building on the modest efforts of earlier workers and continued with studies on his own patients. He supplemented this with what he discovered in a series of novel laboratory experiments. As a district medical officer with initiative and a quest to learn and contribute, he built a foundation that supported the development of the Botox we know today.

Kerner began his work at the age of twenty-nine in Württemberg, Germany, where he was a polymath physician, poet, and philosopher. He excelled in all three during a long and distinguished career that lasted until age seventy-two.[6] In areas of literature, Kerner cofounded the Swabian (related to the medieval German duchy of Swabia or its inhabitants) group of late Romantic poets, and his work was published in the United States.[7,8,9] Symmetrical inkblots he created to inspire poetry evolved into the currently used Rorschach test. In sum, Kerner was described as having that "peculiar work of blending revelations . . . combined with additional confirmatory facts . . . in a strangely novel and romantic form."[10]

In 1822, after more than five years of investigations and having cared for 155 patients with sausage poisoning, Kerner published a summary of his findings from the clinic and laboratory. He blamed a fatty poison in blood sausage that had been consumed by individuals who later experienced illness and death, starting with paralysis of nerves around the eyes, face, and throat. Death, in these cases from respiratory failure, occurred within hours or days. The first task in Kerner's study of causes was to compare the various recipes and ingredients in samples of the sausages he collected. The ingredients included liver, meat, brain, fat, salt, pepper, coriander, pimento, ginger, and bread. The only common findings were blood, salt, and fat. Salt and blood were ruled out as having no significance. Kerner's conclusion was that the harm was caused either by the fat or something it contained.[11]

Next, he conducted experiments on various animals, including birds, cats, rabbits, frogs, flies, locusts, and snails by feeding some with the fatty substance flavored with honey and others with the same material inserted in an incision in the thigh muscle. While the subjects differed greatly, the effect of the fatty material was the same. The creatures that ingested the fatty substance died. In cases where the fat was placed in an incision, the animal survived but the muscle around the fat was weakened. At this point, Kerner concluded that the death-dealing substance from the blood sausage was a biological toxin. After publishing his paper on these results, many began referring to botulism poisoning as *Kerner's disease*. But the most amazing conclusion Justinus Kerner offered from his work was, by way of speculation and theory, based on an unusual experiment.[12]

In a daring move, Kerner placed a dab of the fatty substance on his own tongue. He reported: "Some of the drops of the acid brought onto the tongue caused great drying out of the palette and the pharynx." Kerner deduced that the toxin acted by interrupting nerve signal transmission. Based on this, he predicted that the toxin could be useful as a medicine in cases of drooling and hypersecretion of mucus. In his words: "By analogy it can be expected that in outbreaks of sweat, perhaps also in mucus hypersecretion, the fatty acid will be of therapeutic value." To avoid being guilty of overstatement, Kerner concluded: "What is said here about the fatty acid as a therapeutic drug belongs to the realm of hypothesis and may be confirmed or disproved by observations in the future."[13]

THE MEN WHO FOLLOWED KERNER

After Justinus Kerner's initial burst of discovery, there remained much that needed to be added to the story of botulinum toxin, and several scientists stepped up to make those additions. The next person to accomplish a breakthrough was Émile Pierre-Marie van Ermengem. Between 1895 and 1897, he identified and characterized the bacteria known as *Clostridium botulinum* and confirmed it produced a deadly exotoxin that caused sausage poisoning, now called *botulism*. In 1926, Hermann Sommer isolated a crude form of the toxin. Between 1943 and 1947, at Camp Detrick, Carl Lamanna and his team isolated the pure crystalline botulinum toxin type A, and Arthur Guyton developed a theory about how it affected nerve transmission. After this, using pure toxin from Lamanna, Edward Schantz perfected the culture and assay technique that kept the toxin going. Building on this, scientists like Arnold Burgen, Vernon Brooks, and Daniel Drachman employed the toxin supplied by Schantz in their own laboratories and added new information about its workings. The contributions of these men will assume an important place as the story of the toxin moves forward.

Justinus Kerner carried out his work and assumed his role as the first voice to explain the toxin to patients. The men who followed Kerner excelled at dealing with the bacterium and its toxin. They produced results that unlocked mysteries and paved the way for progress. A summation of all this work set the stage for Alan Scott, who pursued a multiphase effort on the scale of Kerner, as he reintroduced the patient to the story and turned the toxin into a useful drug. Scott worked each morning in a small laboratory supported by minimal funds he raised to support his research. In the afternoon, he cared for patients in his private office. Working on his own, Alan Scott developed a blockbuster drug, succeeding against all odds, as he created a story that deserves telling.

2

The World's Deadliest Poison

Bacteria, toxin, and poison—oh, my!

Why do we need to know about bacteria? That is a legitimate question! To start, we cohabitate with bacteria that are constantly on and in our bodies. Some bacteria deliver disease while others support health and well-being. We need the good ones and survive the troublemakers; but if we meet up with the wrong one and it gets the upper hand, it might kill us. Learning about bacteria at the most basic level, some believe, pales to understanding the dashboard of a new car or managing our cell phones—but we do it.

In the human body, bacteria cells outnumber human cells by a small margin. However, the bacteria we have are tiny. If we could measure, only a scant portion of our body weight would be lost if all the bacteria went away.[1] However, that is not a good idea. Studies have shown that bacteria-free animals don't do well. That goes for humans too. The "good" bacterial flora in our system, like *Lactobacillus*, make it possible for us to digest foods like milk and ice cream. They, and other bacteria called *probiotics*, are quietly doing good things to keep us healthy and happy.[2]

Some bacteria that could be harmful are also with us but are kept at bay by natural processes. For example, *Staphylococcus* in the tear film is removed quickly by blinking or being flushed away in our tears. In a similar way, bacteria on the move, including spores in the gut, may not have time to release a deadly toxin. Potentially harmful bacteria on our skin rarely are around long enough to cause harm and can be washed off before spreading to others—a good reason for frequent handwashing.

In the world of bacteria, there are the good guys and the bad guys. The good guys keep us healthy, like the digestive probiotics, and we tend to take them for granted. The bad guys, like *Staphylococcus aureus*, *Escherichia coli*, *Streptococcus pneumoniae*, and *Salmonella*, are not likely to cause harm on the skin and outside the body. They can, however, cause serious harm if they enter the bloodstream through cuts on the skin or if they invade the digestive system. When these bacteria become established and multiply, an infection can develop in tissues, muscles, nerves, fat, and blood cells. Most can be treated if caught early. Many bad bacteria cause us misery by making us feel unwell for short periods. Fortunately, with time and proper care, we get over it. Some of these can make us sick enough to die from damage to tissue or systemic complications, or kill us outright by producing a separate toxin that has a uniquely harmful effect. Good hygiene, safe food practices, a healthy immune system, and a wide array of antibiotics are a bulwark against harm from most bacteria.

Clostridium Botulinum

Clostridium botulinum is a bacterium that produces the world's most lethal toxin. It has been with us as long as there has been life on earth, but the disease it causes was not recognized in humans until the late 1700s in southern Germany, where it caused sickness and death in groups of otherwise healthy people. It struck suddenly and affected clusters of victims, creating what were described as epidemics. At first, all that was known about this affliction was that it occurred in people who had eaten tainted blood sausage.[3]

A breakthrough in understanding the disease, now called *botulism poisoning* (after *botulus*, the Latin word for *sausage*), occurred in 1895. A group of twenty-three musicians had performed at the funeral of a prominent citizen in Ellezelles, Belgium, and attended a dinner celebration afterward, a common practice. Ham that had been salted and soaked in brine was served. In a few hours, seventeen were hospitalized. All those sickened had eaten the ham. None who had refrained from eating ham became ill. The affected individuals suffered from intestinal discomfort, weakness, droopy eyelids, blurred vision, difficulty swallowing, and shortness of breath that worsened over the next several days. Three of the musicians died.

Professor Émile Pierre-Marie van Ermengem, a bacteriologist at the University of Ghent and the most qualified person to study this outbreak, was summoned. The professor, then age forty-four, had studied in Germany with the famed bacteriologist Robert Koch, who only a decade earlier had discovered the *tubercle bacillus*, the bacterium that causes tuberculosis and was considered the nineteenth century's biggest killer. Along with Louis Pasteur, Koch was considered preeminent in the field of bacteriology. Professor van Ermengem found the bacteria in the ham *and* in the men who had died. He confirmed it as the cause of their poisoning, fulfilling Koch's four postulates:

1. The bacteria must be present in every case of the disease.
2. The bacteria must be isolated from the host with the disease and grown in pure culture.
3. The specific disease must be reproduced when a pure culture of the bacteria is inoculated into a healthy susceptible host.[4]
4. The bacteria must be recoverable from the experimentally infected host.[5]

Bacteria are ubiquitous, and there are about thirty thousand formally named species.[6] Bacteria are mostly free-living organisms consisting of one biological cell without a nucleus but with DNA for replication and expression. Bacteria are typically a few micrometers in length. They are small but can be seen readily and studied using a light microscope in the laboratory with 400× magnification. Bacteria were among the first forms to appear on earth and are present in and on us. They are part of who we are!

At first glance, *Clostridium botulinum* does not appear especially noteworthy. It looks like a hundred other bacteria, and its biological characteristics are for the most part unremarkable. These bacteria are gram-positive rods, spore-forming, anaerobic, and produce a toxin. The key element here is no small thing: the toxin it produces is the most lethal known, and its discovery was hastened by its death-dealing characteristic.[7]

Clostridium botulinum and its toxin have a complicated relationship with the human body. The intact spore can be ingested, and many people probably do so daily without suffering harm. But the spore can become deadly when it dissolves outside the body, allowing the bacteria to form the toxin. When the toxin is ingested and reaches the bloodstream, it immediately blocks the release of acetylcholine at nerve endings, shutting down vital functions including breathing, leading to death, depending on the time and dose. If the spore enters the gut intact, it will pass through the normal adult digestive system harmlessly, not producing the toxin. However, in the infant gut (under one year old) or when embedded deeply in a wound in a prolonged oxygen-free environment, a spore can persist long enough to allow toxin production. It can also be delivered by injection under the skin with a dirty needle.

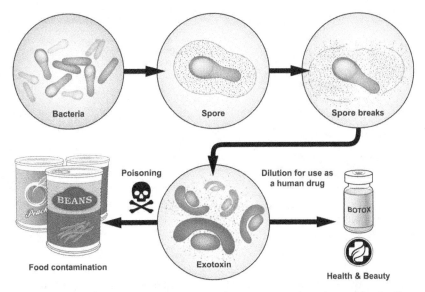

(a) The bacterium *Clostridium botulinum* (b) produces a spore (c) that releases (d) a deadly exotoxin (e). Undiluted, the toxin is death dealing. (f) Diluted, it can provide health and well-being.

Behavior of the Bacteria In Vivo

Bacteria like *Clostridium botulinum* are living cells found in, on, or outside the human body, while viruses are nonliving molecules that depend on a host to reproduce, although they can survive briefly without a host.

Clostridium botulinum bacteria are present worldwide in soil and sediment.

- The bacterial growth thrives in an environment that lacks oxygen (anaerobic).
- In a suitable environment, the number of bacteria can double every twenty minutes and billions could be present in hours.
- Grows best in warm, room temperatures 35 to 37 degrees Celsius—approximately 95 to 110 degrees Fahrenheit.
- Needs a low-salt and low-acid environment to sustain growth (high salt content slows bacteria growth but does not affect toxin).
- Forms a deadly exotoxin (meaning toxin is secreted without destroying the cell).

And there is a zinger: when encountering a hostile environment, the bacteria can form a spore that provides a durable protective coat allowing the bacteria to survive in unfavorable circumstances. Spores (and any

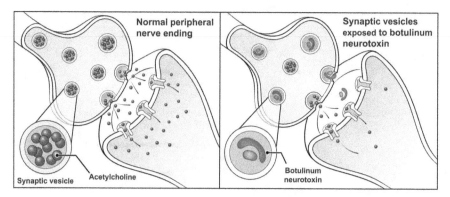

Acetylcholine is produced in the nerve endings and joins the muscle creating muscle contraction (a) botulinum toxin stops acetylcholine production necessary for muscle contraction causing weakness and paralysis (b).

toxin present) are killed by heating to 121 degrees Celsius for ten minutes (approximately 240 degrees Fahrenheit) in a pressure cooker. This is crucial in any canning process.

When conditions become favorable for duplication, the spore breaks and is able to secrete the toxin, defined as a poison or venom produced by bacteria, plant, or animal microorganism. (Think of the toxin you may have encountered from poison ivy, the tip of a yucca plant, *Salmonella*, typhoid toxin, and more.)

Botulinum toxin is colorless and tasteless. As little as eight grams—an amount equal in weight to a lead pencil or three teaspoons of flour—could bring death to the entire population of the world if it were distributed evenly. This toxin is destroyed with around five minutes of heating at 85 degrees Celsius (approximately 185 degrees Fahrenheit).

An undiluted toxin produced by the spore-forming bacteria is lethal in doses as small as billionths of a gram. The most common spread is via food where proper precautions have been neglected, especially in food canned without proper heating. It can also be found in food that has been heated or refrigerated and then left at room temperature for long periods, enough to allow for cell numbers to increase and produce the toxin.

Diluted to tenths of billionths of a gram, botulinum toxin can be administered to a human safely. Since 1989, it has been employed as a medicine for health and cosmetic purposes, fulfilling Paracelsus's dictum: "All things are poison. Only the dose determines a thing is not a poison."

Once the ingested toxin is delivered into the blood, it targets the nerve endings that secrete acetylcholine, a necessary substance for transmitting the impulse from the nerve ending to the muscle or to another structure re-sponding to the nerve, like a sweat gland.[8] The more toxin present, the more nerve impulses are blocked and the more deadly the toxin's effect. The in-dividual structures normally secreting acetylcholine are not destroyed, just deactivated—temporarily disabled. In weeks to months, the disabled secre-tory structures in the nerve endings begin to regain the ability to secrete acetylcholine, restoring nerve function. If the patient survives the acute phase, everything is back to normal within weeks to months. Toxin circu-lating in the blood that has not reached the nerve ending can be destroyed by equine botulinum antitoxin. Protective antibodies can be produced by the body ahead of time by use of a vaccine.

Toxin Effect in Humans

Clostridium botulinum can enter the body ingested with food in two forms: either as a potentially toxin-forming spore or as an already formed toxin. Spores that enter the digestive tract pass through without breaking and re-leasing the bacteria capable of secreting toxin. This passage of *Clostridium*

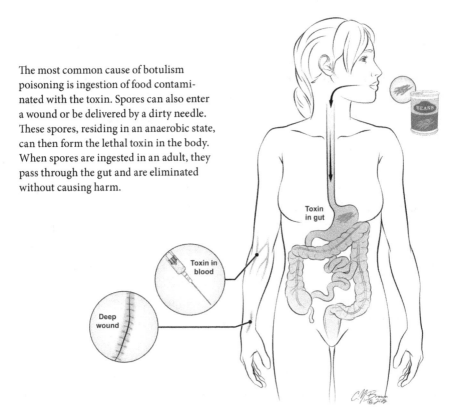

The most common cause of botulism poisoning is ingestion of food contami-nated with the toxin. Spores can also enter a wound or be delivered by a dirty needle. These spores, residing in an anaerobic state, can then form the lethal toxin in the body. When spores are ingested in an adult, they pass through the gut and are eliminated without causing harm.

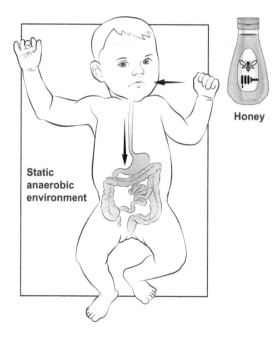

Honey

Static anaerobic environment

Infant botulism poisoning occurs when spores form the toxin in the slow-moving gut of a child under one year old. Infants should not be fed honey, a food that contains abundant spores.

botulinum spores through the gut could be an everyday occurrence for some.

Wound botulism occurs when spores enter a wound or are introduced under the skin with a dirty needle. These spores in the depth of the wound, which is an anaerobic environment, can remain long enough to release bacteria that produce toxin, resulting in botulism poisoning when the toxin is absorbed in the bloodstream.

Infant botulism poisoning, first discovered in 1976, accounts for 75 percent of botulism poisoning now seen in the United States. Mortality in infant botulism is now near zero. A rule for children under a year old, especially six months and younger, is that they should not be fed honey, which is likely to contain *Clostridium botulinum* spores. In an infant less than a year old, spores can remain in the gut long enough to release bacteria that can produce toxin in the body. When toxin forms, it enters the infant's bloodstream and affects the nervous system, producing what has been described as a "floppy baby."[9]

HOW THE BACTERIA AND ITS TOXIN BEHAVE

Clostridium botulinum is found in soil and sediment throughout the world. There is no known way to alter its behavior in a natural setting other than destroying the organism or deactivating the potentially death-dealing toxin molecule. The best defense is to discourage its propagation by paying attention to the requirements for growth of any bacteria in the foods you ingest and to avoid the use of dirty needles. A simple mnemonic has been offered to assist as a reminder of our best strategy for protecting against any bacteria, including *Clostridium botulinum*. The mnemonic is FATTOM.[10]

F is for food and is a reminder that the bacterium needs some type of protein substrate to continue growing. This substrate turns out to be many meats, fish, eggs, and a variety of low-acid vegetables. So many are included, it is virtually impossible to avoid enough foods to be able to say you are free of any chance for botulism poisoning.

A is for acid. *Clostridium botulinum* does not grow in a strongly acidic environment. That means it is more likely to increase with a higher pH, usually above 4.5. This is still acidic but less so.

T is for temperature, which is crucial when dealing with *Clostridium botulinum*. A temperature of 185 degrees Fahrenheit for 15 minutes will neutralize all the toxin, and 240-plus degrees Fahrenheit for ten minutes in a pressure cooker will eliminate all spores. This also could be a reminder that other temperatures, like high room temperatures along with low oxygen, can contribute to cell replication and toxin formation. Foods eaten directly without heating can be especially dangerous. Food should not be left standing at room temperature but should be refrigerated until serving cold or being reheated.

T is for time, which is also key. Since the number of bacteria can double every twenty minutes, a food that contains bacteria and is producing toxin will become more dangerous with time. Don't allow foods to linger at room temperature. Store them in a refrigerator and heat them thoroughly before eating. Do not let food stand to attain room temperature before putting it in the refrigerator. This was done when we "cooled" foods in the icebox. The practice was intended to make the cooling blocks of ice last longer, not to protect food. It is outdated and could be dangerous.

O is for oxygen—or rather, its absence, which is necessary for the growth of *Clostridium botulinum* and the production of its lethal toxin. Paradoxically, the beneficial effects of food preservation in canning offer a perfect environment for the growth of botulinum toxin if the food is canned without proper preheating to kill the spores. If spores are included in the anaerobic atmosphere of a canned food with moisture, it is a perfect place to produce toxin or retain toxin that is already present. Current commercial canning practice virtually eliminates this.

M is for moisture, a necessary ingredient for the growth of toxin-forming *Clostridium botulinum*. Spores can survive in a dry environment, but they do not release bacteria that can replicate and form toxin until a moist environment is restored.

DANGERS OF THE TOXIN

Botulinum toxin has no odor, color, or taste. While these features might cause the toxin to be less unpleasant initially, they also render it potentially more dangerous. Food tainted with botulinum toxin will not send up a red flag to suggest some form of danger to the unsuspecting. This contrasts with other types of spoiled food that would be unappetizing and therefore not likely to be eaten. Moreover, the toxin has no effect on your sensory system. It does not diminish smell, taste, or visual acuity, nor does it affect cognition.

Furthermore, there is virtually no way to absolutely safeguard yourself from ever having botulism poisoning. Fortunately, the disease is rare because of excellent food management systems that are in effect worldwide in developed countries. In addition, the environment required for toxin formation is exacting. That is, everything must be in line and be just so for the toxin to be produced. And even if (more likely when) a human ingests spores, it is extremely unlikely to result in that person developing botulism poisoning. In the normal adult digestion process, there is insufficient time for the spores to colonize and produce toxin before being eliminated. Adult colonization botulism poisoning is so rare it is hardly worth mentioning.

BOTULISM POISONING

Foodborne botulism occurs when an adult ingests food where toxin has already formed. Outbreaks of botulism poisoning have been reported in groups that have eaten the same food at an event where home-canned and prepared foods that already contain toxin are served. In these cases, it is usually possible to isolate the source by testing the food that is left over. This can be confirmed by noting that all who ate that food have been affected and all who avoided that food are free of symptoms.[11]

The symptoms of botulism poisoning are said to begin with what is called a *descending paralysis*. It starts at the "top," or the head, affecting the cranial nerves causing drooping eyelids, double vision, dilated pupils, and blurred near vision. From there, weakness affects swallowing, speech, and produces a dry throat. These symptoms are caused initially by disruption of

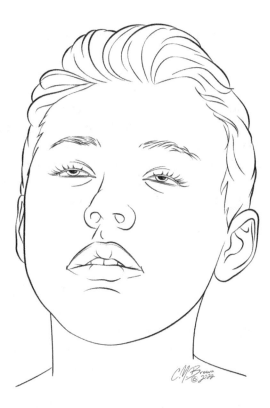

The descending paralysis of botulism poisoning starts with dilated pupils, drooping of the upper lids, and a dull, expressionless face.

the autonomic nervous system. That is the part of the nervous system that is always functioning and is not dependent on being told what to do.

We don't tell our pupils to dilate when it is dark or constrict in bright light. Likewise, functions such as swallowing, salivation, and even aspects of breathing are in effect on "automatic pilot." The autonomic nervous system being affected is like having the plumbing in a building turned off. All the various functions dealing with supply and drainage of water served by plumbing would eventually be affected. These would include hot water, cold water, flushing the toilet, adding water to a humidifier, draining the bathtub, and so on. Described as a descending paralysis, it means weakness from botulism poisoning starts at the top, and when it gets about halfway down and includes your lungs, breathing stops and that can be the end. Respiratory paralysis is the most common cause of death in botulism poisoning.

Other muscles that run on a voluntary system and respond based on intention, or that serve other functions, like sweating, are usually affected later. When this happens, there can be weakness of the limbs, along with lower-body autonomic system involvement, like reduced intestinal motility causing stomach upset and constipation. Emptying the bladder can also be affected and require catheterization.

Many of the later-appearing symptoms of botulism poisoning may never be seen because with a lethal dose of the toxin, death from respiratory failure occurs before other warning signs are evident. More distant problems like constipation, urinary retention, loss of sweating, and others are more likely to occur in milder or survivable protracted cases. These are the kind that would result from smaller doses of the toxin or in a patient who survives after timely initial treatment.

Affecting the Nervous System

When the toxin enters the bloodstream, it enables the toxin-laden blood to reach the nerve endings responsible for sending the nerve stimulus on to or toward the responding muscle. In the autonomic nervous system, this happens at the first junction and affects all the functions downstream from there. These are the first systems to fail. Other muscles, including those that are voluntary, are affected when the toxin acts at the junction of the nerve directly affecting the muscle.

In both cases, the toxin enters the end of the nerve and obstructs the pores of discrete structures that deliver a substance called *acetylcholine*. This is the substance that must be present for the nerve impulse to be delivered to the muscle that will eventually contract.

There are many redundant structures, or units, in the nerve ending capable of sending the acetylcholine message, and it takes one toxin molecule to stop one unit. A small amount of toxin causes a little weakness, but with a sufficiently large amount of toxin, a major shutdown of the nerve signal occurs, resulting in stoppage of these signals, loss of muscle contraction, and death usually when breathing stops!

This disruption in the supply of acetylcholine is like when the plug on a lamp cord is corroded by rust.[12] The lamp will only light up if the electricity can get to it. The problem is the two perfectly normal constituents are not functioning simply because their connection is blocked. The toxin can stop the acetylcholine supply for three or four months. After this time, the structures that release the connecting substance, acetylcholine, are restored to normal, and in the patient that survives there is no residual effect except for whatever conditioning was lost during the forced inactivity. The dose-related effect in a drug like Botox, with a wide range of safety along with the natural reversibility of the toxin's effect, should be reassuring to those who undergo botulinum toxin (Botox) treatment on an elective basis because a "bad" result is only temporary.

Now a little more on the "good" side in terms of botulinum toxin being a useful medicine. Botulinum toxin is powerful, and this power can be accurately measured by regular assays of the culture in a lab. When the toxin is diluted to the appropriate strength, stabilized, freeze-dried, and placed in a vial for reconstitution, the dosage remains stable. The toxin can be diluted sufficiently to achieve a dosage that is both safe and effective. Even a large therapeutic dose, which could be two hundred units—the total contents of two vials—can be as little as *one fifteenth* the amount that would be fatal to a human.[13] Moreover, there appears to be little variation in how patients react to botulinum toxin treatment. Results from toxin injection depend on the dose. The outcome is consistent, meaning similar doses tend to produce similar results, which should be reassuring for the patient! Botulinum toxin type A is very nearly the perfect fulfillment of Paracelsus's dictum from the sixteenth century: "What is there that is not poison? All things are poison, and nothing is without poison. Solely the dose determines that a thing is not a poison."[14]

Based mostly on Kerner's and van Ermengem's work, the causes of botulism poisoning were well understood by the end of the nineteenth century. However, another food-related activity that started in France around the time of Kerner's discoveries would set the stage for outbreaks of botulism poisoning in the United States after the turn of the twentieth century. These were closely associated with a new technique for food preservation, canning, which was being carried out on a commercial basis. The widespread distribution of foods produced without stringent processing guidelines spelled trouble. This called for an accelerated scientific process that would result in a better understanding of the bacterium and how to control it to make sure our food was safe.

3

The Canning Industry

Canning brought nourishment to millions of people, but it also provided the perfect environment for Clostridium botulinum and its toxin.

A round the beginning of the nineteenth century, the issue of providing safe, wholesome food to city dwellers and nourishing food to the army in the field was at the forefront—and a solution was sought. Two important characters who answered the call to action were a general who later became the head of the French government and a French chef. Between them, the canning industry got its start.

The canning process, as a means of preserving food, originated in the last decade of the eighteenth century in France. This notion was spurred by Napoleon, who was dismayed when he saw his troops suffer from scurvy and other conditions that he felt were the result of a poor diet. To remedy this situation, General Bonaparte sought a better way to provide wholesome meals for his troops fighting far from home. As more forces were deployed, this became a matter of national concern. Searching for a solution, the French government offered a prize of 12,000 francs (equivalent to about ten years of median income at the time) for the person who could deliver a process that would provide safe and healthful food.

Nicolas Appert, a Frenchman skilled in brewing, distilling, and confectionery, had developed such a process in the 1790s.[1] His method for preserving food was to place a vegetable, fruit, or meat into a glass bottle that he sealed with a cork held in place by wire. The bottles were placed in boiling water for varying times depending on the food and were subsequently allowed to cool. These bottles of prepared food were initially provided to the French Navy. To the sailors' delight, the contents were still good three months later. (The words *can* and *canning* are a derivation of the word *cannister*, which described the bottles used.) When Appert reported his success, he was awarded the 12,000-franc prize. Napoleon, who is credited with the saying "An army marches on its stomach" was influential at the start of the canning industry, and this comment supports that claim.[2]

The use of canned food was not limited to the military. It was enjoyed in affluent households by families who were now beginning to experience this benefit. Soon the idea of producing canned food spread to Britain and finally to the United States. Two notable front-runners that are still in business today are Heinz and Campbell.

Dealing with another staple, Gail Borden developed a process to condense and preserve milk produced in the nation's first canned milk plant. Over the century, techniques improved, and the canning industry increased in size. The variety of canned products, starting with ketchup and soup, expanded from a few to many, along with widespread distribution. This eventually called for the establishment of standards and safety measures to protect consumers.[3]

RULES FOR FOOD SAFETY

With the start of the twentieth century, the United States experienced the assassination of its newly reelected president. On September 6, 1901, William McKinley was shot and killed during a visit to Buffalo, New York. President McKinley had planned to join the citizens of Buffalo to celebrate the opening of the Pan-American Exposition. He was scheduled to meet the public at the Temple of Music theater, where he would spend two hours shaking hands. A long line of well-wishers had assembled in advance of the 4:00 p.m. start time. They were eager to meet President McKinley, who was known for the approachability he had demonstrated four years earlier during his front porch campaign in Ohio. Just minutes into the event, a twenty-eight-year-old man, who was an avowed anarchist, shot the president twice with a .32-caliber revolver. The man later said, "All those people seemed bowing to the great ruler. I made up my mind to kill that ruler."[4]

The fifty-eight-year-old McKinley, the most popular president in decades, had been greeted the night before with pyrotechnics that spelled out "Welcome President McKinley, Chief of Our Nation and Our Empire." Did those grandiose words spur on his killer? President McKinley died from complications of his wounds eight days later. McKinley's untimely death led to a series of events that would result in the promotion of food safety in the United States. The office of president was filled by forty-two-year-old Vice President Theodore Roosevelt. Young Roosevelt had been placed on the ticket for McKinley's second term because his first vice president, Garrett Hobart, had died in office in 1899, two years before, and the position had not been filled.

The new president assumed office as a Republican full of progressive ideas. One of Roosevelt's strategies was to enlist the aid of Harvey W. Wiley, head of the chemistry division of the Agriculture Department.[5] Roosevelt's aim was to establish policies to ensure the population was provided food that was both safe and free of adulteration with harmful additives. Efforts of this pair led Congress to establish the Pure Food and Drug Act of 1906, which was the forerunner of today's Food and Drug Administration. There was wide support for this legislation, which would also be effective in curbing abuses that were becoming rampant in the meat-processing industry.

The president and the director had slightly different trajectories that diverged widely at times. Wiley focused on ridding food of substances he believed were adulterations, calling them deleterious and dangerous ingredients. For him, these ingredients included additives like sugar and caffeine—things the president liked.

Zealously pursuing his aims, Wiley took on Coca-Cola and Heinz, decrying their use of these ingredients and demanding they stop. He was unsuccessful in both cases, as attested by a trip to the supermarket today. The president's aim was to improve sanitation and safety in the food industry by establishing and enforcing new standards. Roosevelt worked closely with big businesses, which in turn supported his efforts. Each recognized that neither would be successful working alone. President Roosevelt believed there was a role for the government in establishing guidelines and to serve as a watchdog, but success depended on cooperation from industry—nothing was more important than food.

The president's interest in food safety may have been driven by his experience leading troops in the Spanish-American War. Thousands of soldiers, whom he led only a few years earlier, were made sick; many died from eating the food that was provided, including canned meat sold by the meatpacking companies, Swift & Company and Armour & Company. In this conflict, more troops died from food poisoning than from combat! No detailed records are available, but the deaths of troops who subsisted on a diet of canned food raises the possibility that some of these deaths could have been from botulism poisoning.[6]

In 1906, Upton Sinclair exposed abuses in the meatpacking industry in his novel *The Jungle*, set in Chicago, then the hub of US meatpacking. This could have pulled off the scab for the sensitized president. In characterizing the events of the book, Roosevelt compared the squalid conditions associated with the meatpackers as *muck* and the antagonist author as *raking the mess* into a pile. Sinclair was the *muckraker* in a word that was added to the vocabulary. With this, the term *muckraking* was defined as "searching out and publicizing scandalous information."[7]

With the advent of canning to process food, a question lurked but there was no one to ask it: how would *Clostridium botulinum* affect the burgeoning canning industry? Did this new process provide safer food? Is that why no outbreaks of botulism poisoning were reported in the nineteenth century in the United States? Or were people dying from botulism poisoning that went unrecognized because the condition was not well known? After all, it was just surfacing as a problem in Germany. There were no ready answers.

There is no evidence that practices were better in the United States, although they may have been different. As for overlooking botulism poisoning, that is unlikely because the pattern of outbreaks is to affect people who have dined in groups—like families or community gatherings—in a way that would call attention. The best answer to these questions might be that neither one is completely right nor completely wrong. Despite a rise in the number of canned foods consumed in the United States, evidence of botulism poisoning reported in the nineteenth century is lacking.

A possible explanation for there being no ready evidence of recorded botulism deaths in the United States during that period is that while canning was practiced, it was not widespread. Instead, food was prepared fresh, mostly heated, and probably eaten promptly. If the food was stored, it was salted and protected against *Clostridium botulinum*. Moreover, it is also possible in that era that cause of death was not determined accurately or recorded precisely.[8]

Early canned foods were often mushy and unappetizing. Though safe, these foods could be unappealing and therefore not sought after. An exception was the California olive, which looked especially appealing, even beautiful, stacked in narrow glass bottles for consumers to enjoy seeing before tasting. But this display's allure proved to be potentially fatal.

When it came to common foods in the United States, there was no known American counterpart to the blood sausage being consumed in southern Germany. This unique food required extensive preparation, relied on multiple ingredients, and most likely spent a fair amount of time lingering at room temperature, with components deeply embedded in an anaerobic environment before the sausage was eaten—conducive to the growth of bacteria and the formation of toxin.

In the nineteenth century and the beginning of the twentieth century, food was cooled with iceboxes and the practice of saving food was not likely to be carried out widely. Food was consumed soon after preparation. *Clostridium botulinum* was doubtless present in the United States, but long-term food storage via the common practice of drying and salting discouraged growth of the bacteria, which preferred a moist, low-salt environment for production of its lethal toxin. Food was prepared fresh, and pictures of old kitchens with wood stoves, cooking fireplaces, and campfires outside suggest food was served hot and eaten promptly and completely! Even if food containing *Clostridium botulinum* spores was ingested, the spores would not remain in the system long enough for toxin to form. This meant people would not be at risk for botulism poisoning.

GUARDING AGAINST *CLOSTRIDIUM BOTULINUM*

With the advent of widespread commercial canning, which employed airtight, sealed cans or glass bottles, one requirement for the formulation of toxin was present: the absence of oxygen. Moreover, in the canning process, moist food is often stored for long periods at room temperature, an environment suitable to increase the number of bacteria. These conditions are ideal for bacteria to grow and eventually form toxin. This sounds like a doomsday scenario, but there is a solution: heat and time.

Today, commercial canners process food at high temperatures, 240 degrees Fahrenheit under pressure for ten minutes, which is a sufficient time to destroy any toxin present and kill *all* bacteria and spores. Home canners are instructed to heat the canning jars according to strict guidelines. A common recommendation for home canning is to heat the jars, filled with the prepared food and sealed, in a pressure cooker for ten minutes or longer, achieving the same temperature as commercial food processors. However, there are variations and anyone planning to be a home canner should follow best practices.[9]

4

An Outbreak in the United States

*Canned black olives from California cause outbreaks of
death in the Midwest and eastern United States.*

The ingredients for a botulinum toxin epidemic were in place in the United States at the turn of the twentieth century. Commercial canning was becoming widespread, but specific guidelines for safety had not been formalized. Those that were in place were unevenly drawn and the mechanism was not yet established to ensure compliance. It seemed only a matter of time before problems would arise.[1]

A deadly outbreak of botulism poisoning that was widely publicized and thoroughly studied occurred in the United States in 1919 and 1920.[2] The origin was canned black olives from California. People who were affected lived throughout the West, Midwest, and East. Half of the victims lived in Ohio and Michigan, where the outbreaks were the most thoroughly studied. The olives were shipped nationwide, and the broad reach from a common source spelled trouble. An irony in this story is that the first episode of this botulism outbreak occurred in the city where President William McKinley was buried.

The epicenter, and thoroughly studied outbreak, of foodborne botulism poisoning in the United States occurred in August 1919 in Canton, Ohio. Similar outbreaks took place in the same month in three other states: Michigan, Montana, and Tennessee. A tragic outbreak of botulism poisoning that virtually wiped out an entire family occurred a few months later in New York City. The offending food in each case was black olives that were grown, processed, and packed in California. Black "ripe" olives were picked green and processed to achieve "forced" ripening to make them different from tree-ripened olives, or genetically black olives that are mostly mottled.

The processing included soaking the olives in lye, followed by washing and aeration that eventually produced an anaerobic environment conducive to the formation of *Clostridium botulinum* spores and toxin. These were not destroyed in the canning process; the glass containers that were used could not withstand a temperature high enough to kill the toxin and spores.

The Banquet in Canton

On August 23, 1919, at a banquet held at the Lakeside Country Club in Canton, Ohio, more than two hundred guests attended and seven died within days, suffering the same symptoms. The dinner served included cantaloupe, turkey, turkey stuffing, tomatoes and mayonnaise, crackers, scalloped corn and pimentos, brown potatoes, green olives, celery and pickles, rolls, butter, ice cream, cake, water, and coffee. However, there was an exception.[3]

Two tables hosted by Helen Sebring Gahris omitted the green olives, celery, and pickles. Instead, her guests were served nuts, candy, and a dish of black olives. Mrs. Gahris purchased the olives at a grocery in Alliance, Ohio, a small town near Canton. Her guests, in addition to the hostess and her husband, included a dozen of the most prominent businessmen and professionals and their wives. A special guest was a local hero from the recently completed Great War. A gala event was planned.

Of the fourteen people seated at the two tables Mrs. Gahris hosted, all had eaten the olives and became sick. Five eventually died. Their deaths occurred within five to seventy hours. In addition, a waiter who ate five or six olives died after fifty-four hours, and the chef who ate two olives died after seventy-five hours—resulting in a death toll of seven. The nine other guests at the Gahris tables and another waiter became ill, but they survived.

The public health officer charged with investigating the cause of the deaths was Charles Armstrong. He was a thirty-three-year-old physician and scientist who worked with the Office of the Surgeon General. He meticulously recorded the events surrounding this outbreak and the result of his investigation was conclusive.

Doctor Armstrong's expertise in epidemiology had been honed by his work in the fight against the worldwide influenza epidemic that occurred during World War I. After Armstrong completed his work there, the US surgeon general ordered him to return to his home state of Ohio on July 1, 1919—just six weeks before the country club banquet. It was a stroke of luck that this brilliant young scientist was the one to assist state health officers, according to his orders, "in any way he could." Armstrong's first assignment was to take charge of the investigation of these deaths. He was hardworking, ambitious, and skilled at his job. (Later he discovered a virus he named *lymphocytic choriomeningitis mammarenavirus*, which led to him gaining worldwide recognition for the important role his discovery of this virus played in the development of the polio vaccine.[4])

Doctor Armstrong conducted interviews with other guests at the banquet and completed a thorough epidemiological study of all the menu items that were still available. They were tested for the presence of *Clostridium botulinum* and its toxin. None was found to be contaminated. Armstrong, by a process of elimination, reasoned that only a food that contained the toxin could be responsible for the deaths and it must have been served at Garris's tables! In a brilliant piece of detective work, Armstrong concluded that the *only* common thread in these deaths was the ingestion of black olives. No guest who had not eaten one of these olives became ill. All those who ate these olives became ill or died. The only variable resulting in sickness was eating a black olive, and the only common thread in not becoming ill or dying was *not* eating one. All the evidence was circumstantial because no olives from the Canton outbreak remained. Later in the investigations of the other outbreaks tied to the same source as those purchased in Ohio, black olives that contained botulinum toxin were recovered.

Armstrong was shown the jar that had contained the olives. It was designed to be vacuum sealed. The kitchen staff told him the lid came off easily without having to be punctured or requiring the use of an instrument. This suggested the seal had been broken. The lid itself was discarded but the recovered glass jar was not cracked or defective in any way. Since *Clostridium botulinum* is anaerobic, the loose cover that could have admitted oxygen played no role. The bacteria and toxin were introduced with the olives when they were packed. The death-dealing toxin was already in the bottle at the time of purchase.

One of the waiters who ate several olives was reported to have said they did not taste right. He wanted to get another opinion, so he gave two olives to the chef, who ate both. The waiter and the chef both died within days. Another waiter had reported this information. He also admitted to eating several olives himself. With a wink he said, "Perhaps the amount of whiskey I drank saved me from dying." A similar comment was made by one of the surviving guests at a Gahris table. Consistent among those who ate the olives and survived was that they "bit the tongue" and "stuck to the tongue." They were just "not fit to eat." Some said they were "soft."[5]

Days after the seven deaths in Canton, seven people died after eating black olives at a dinner party in Grosse Pointe, Michigan. Alerted by the events in Ohio, doctors were able to recover *Clostridium botulinum* from the olives served. Brine from the Michigan bottle containing the olives was injected into a laboratory mouse and proved to be fatal, confirming the presence of the lethal toxin. This supported the presumptive diagnosis in the Ohio deaths. Later evidence confirmed the olives consumed in both Michigan and Ohio were packed on the same day and in the same plant in California. Less is known about the deaths that occurred at this time in two other states: Tennessee and Montana.

STILL MORE DEATH

Another tragic olive-related event took place a few months later. It started on the evening of January 9, 1920, when a thirty-three-year-old woman in the Bronx became ill suddenly. Her problems started with vomiting. "She spent the night weeping and worrying over increasingly disturbing symptoms." In the morning, complaining of difficulty swallowing and blurred vision, she had trouble speaking and "struggled desperately for breath." Her mind was clear, but she was in great distress.[6]

When she told her husband about her breathing difficulty, a physician was called to the home. The doctor found Mrs. Delbene's temperature and reflexes to be normal. Finding nothing amiss beyond the woman's complaint, he told the family to have her rest and call if she continued to have problems. He was called back within an hour. On his arrival, the woman was dead, less than twenty-four hours after the onset of symptoms. He had no answer for the cause of her death. She had been treated earlier for kidney difficulties, so the doctor reported her death to be from chronic nephritis, uremia.

Three days later, the mourning family assembled in their kitchen to prepare a meal. It consisted of macaroni with tomato sauce and a salad made of anchovies, pickled peppers, black olives, olive oil, and vinegar. At this family dinner were the husband, Paul; his two brothers, Dominic and Angelo; two sons, Dominica and Antonio; and his daughter, Lena. The youngest boy, Joe, age seven, was away with relatives. By ten o'clock that evening, the eldest son, Dominica, became ill with symptoms like his mother had three days before. Unbeknownst to them, the family would be reenacting the scene that had taken the life of Mary Delbene. She undoubtedly had sampled the olives that led to her demise. The same olives had been eaten by her surviving family. Within three days, five more family members were dead. There were only two survivors: Lena, who was at the dinner and became ill but survived, and her brother Joe, who was away. By this time, the doctors at the hospital where the family members had been treated were aware of the botulism poisoning from olives in the Midwest earlier.

Epidemiological studies and laboratory tests of the Delbene family pointed conclusively to botulism poisoning from eating California black olives. The olives first snacked on by Mrs. Delbene and later eaten by her family had been tainted with deadly botulism toxin at the time of canning. Health officials later discovered the jar of olives in the Delbene kitchen. They analyzed the remaining olives and found botulinum toxin. A massive effort to remove bottles with the olives from the same consignment was undertaken by New York's health commissioner. The death-dealing California olives in New York were determined to be from a different packer than those that led to deaths in the Midwest. This suggested the problem could be not just local but systemic, potentially affecting any California olive packer.

Where It Started

Olives were on the menu as an appetizer in the finest restaurants as well as in many homes in the United States around the start of the twentieth century. This food, introduced from the Mediterranean region, was becoming popular and was processed locally. In 1774, Thomas Jefferson planted olive stones at Monticello with the aim of olives becoming an important Southern crop.[7] His lifelong efforts were in vain. It took until 1901, in Southern California, for the United States olive industry to find its footing. This effort was led by Professor F. T. Bioletti of the University of California, who is called the "father of the black olive industry." If this industry has a father, it also has a mother: Freda Ehmann, another leader in the field.[8] She moved to California in the 1890s as a widow with no money. Through hard work and with a dream, she pioneered the state's olive industry. The company she formed still bears her name and operates to this day.

The Need for Regulation

After a promising start that resulted in olive sales being carried out nationwide, California's black olive industry was rocked by news of the 1920 epidemic, which included more than two dozen deaths in five states. This prompted efforts on the part of the state and national groups to establish best practices and safe management for the industry. The newly established Hooper Foundation in San Francisco hired Professor Karl Meyer to lead this effort. Working with packers, academics, and the government, his team developed methods for heating and packaging that provided assurance that foods canned with their methods would be safe. Their technique would destroy bacteria and toxin and not harm the food product.[9]

Black olives in glass containers had been heated for shorter periods at lower heat because the glass bottles were not able to withstand the higher temperatures required to kill spores. This resulted in a conundrum. The packers wanted to stick with the glass because they showed off the beauty of their product. Salesmen were provided with these slender glass bottles with perfectly stacked black olives for demonstration to help close the sale. They were overruled by food safety experts, who demanded the use of metal containers able to withstand the higher temperatures necessary to kill spores. Today's consumer will recognize that all black olives that have been processed to achieve "forced ripening" are sold in cans! They are safe.

The State of California endorsed the Cannery Inspection Act of 1925.[10] Both the State Board of Health and the National Canners Association agreed to be sponsors. They also favored federal inspection to make sure that good practices were maintained. Today California's Food and Drug branch inspects two hundred licensed canners dealing with a wide variety of foods where regulated products are packaged. Its primary goal remains maintaining food safety while preventing foodborne botulism.

It appears that the bottom line in food safety for botulism is to heat the food to a sufficient temperature for an appropriate length of time. There are specific regulations for each type of food, but it is only a matter of paying attention to the recipe and carrying it out.

5

A Rare and Deadly Disease

In the twenty-first century, botulism poisoning is rare, affecting about one hundred people in the United States each year. Mortality is 3 percent, and in the most common form—infant botulism poisoning—deaths are under 1 percent. Botox and other commercially available brands of botulinum toxin are used worldwide for health and beauty.

Though rare, the threat of botulism poisoning remains, and there is reason to remain vigilant by continuing safe food practices and maintaining a sense of awareness. Since the 1970s, the facts and clinical guidelines for botulinum toxin are as follows:

- Botulism poisoning, when determined with a presumptive diagnosis, is treated with equine antitoxin within thirty-six hours to neutralize unbound toxin in the bloodstream. The antitoxin is available 24/7 after contacting the state health department or from the Centers for Disease Control and Prevention (CDC) Emergency Operations Center (770-488-7100).
- For infant botulism (floppy baby), human immune globulin is preferred, but equine antitoxin, which is much less expensive, is also successful.
- When toxin enters the bloodstream, within thirty-six hours all of it has engaged with nerve endings to shut down the release of acetylcholine. When this happens, treatment for an affected individual includes a variety of supportive measures in a hospital setting, including the use of a respirator if breathing difficulties develop.
- Timing is key to successful treatment, especially when treating with an antitoxin.
- Food safety measures primarily related to the commercial canning industry are in place based on cooperation between government and private industry. This has virtually eliminated botulism poisoning in commercial canning.
- Home canners are provided with readily available support and guidelines for safe practices, with information and contacts available online.

- Botulism is most likely to result when foods that might contain an otherwise harmless number of spores are inadequately heated or are allowed to remain at room temperature for long periods of time, sufficient for the growth of bacteria and production of toxin before being consumed.
- Botulism poisoning affects about one hundred people per year in the United States, with 75 percent of cases being infants.
- The incidence of death from botulism poisoning is about 3 percent in adults who are affected (compared to 50 percent prior to the mid-twentieth century). Mortality is virtually zero in infants.
- Specially prepared botulinum toxin is on the horizon to treat millions of people worldwide for health and cosmetic indications.
- Botulism caused by using dirty needles is the only type of botulism poisoning likely to be increasing in the United States.

Anyone suffering botulism poisoning today would more likely have an outcome like the story that follows, which is based on a case report in medical literature. The characters are fictional, but this is how a typical scenario would unfold.

Bill and Anne were healthy and in their thirties. They were looking forward to their first meal in their new home after a busy day of moving. For dinner they decided on carryout. When Bill returned from picking up dinner, he announced, "Spaghetti Bolognese, salad, and garlic bread. Oh, and don't forget Mom's salad." Anne's mother had dropped by in the afternoon to deliver her famous three-bean salad, made from a new batch of beans she had canned. Anne knew the dish did not go with the Italian food, but they could at least have a taste and save the rest of the three-bean salad for tomorrow. The couple called their repast "comfort food for a victory banquet," and each made a point of sampling Mom's dish.[1]

Their joy did not last. By the next morning, instead of looking forward to a quiet day in their new apartment, watching the Sunday football game, Anne complained of stomach pain and nausea. When she told Bill how she felt, he realized he was not far from that himself but had decided not to make it a big thing. They had a quiet and unpleasant day.

The following day at 6:30 a.m., Anne felt no better, and by now, Bill admitted he felt rotten too, with the added problem of blurred vision. Both called into work to take a sick day. Hoping to get ahead of whatever was going on with them, Bill decided they should go to the emergency room.

Shortly after arriving and registering, they were directed to a curtained enclosure where the examination would begin. When a nurse entered, Anne made it clear that both she and Bill were patients. Then the two answered routine preliminary questions, starting with telling the nurse why they were there and that their general health was good. Two more questions about allergies and current medications were all the nurse asked. Then she checked their temperature, blood pressure, pulse, and respiration and charted the results for each.

The nurse asked a few final questions. Speaking for both, Anne answered, saying they had eaten their last meal at home Saturday night and since then had eaten almost nothing. She had vomited Sunday morning. When Anne said she had some difficulty swallowing, Bill volunteered, "My vision is blurry, and when I look in the distance, sometimes I see double." With that the nurse left, saying the doctor would be in shortly.

In a few minutes, a smiling, youthful-appearing doctor, attired in blue scrubs and a white lab coat, entered and introduced himself. Before saying more, he looked at the nurse's notes and said, "Anything to add?"

"Not really," said Bill. Then after a pause, he added, "Well, maybe there is a little more. I am a bit dizzy, and I have had trouble swallowing." Except when he said that, it came out "swawoowing."

The doctor noticed Bill's slurred speech. Admitting that *swallowing* is a difficult word to say, he realized the patient had really messed it up. Taking a closer look at both Bill and Anne, he asked, "Have you noticed that your pupils are dilated?"

This caused his patients to look at each other, and in unison they said, "Yes, they are, aren't they?"

The doctor asked the pair to sit on the edge of the examining table and look at him while they forcibly closed their eyes. "Really clamp down your lids and repeat this ten times," he said. When Bill and Anne finished, the doctor noticed both acted as though their lids wanted to stay closed, stuck together. They had to strain to open their eyelids, and even after that effort, the lids of both drooped some.

"When did you eat last?" was the doctor's next question.

Anne spoke, "Actually, it was two days ago, Saturday night. We felt so crummy yesterday and this morning that we ate about nothing."

"What did you eat?"

"Spaghetti Bolognese, tossed salad with Caesar dressing, a bit of bean salad, and garlic bread," offered Bill.

"Was that all?"

"Oh, and a glass of Chianti."

"Did all the food come from the same place?"

"No," said Anne. "The spaghetti, salad, and bread were carryout from a restaurant, and the few bites of bean salad were from my mother. That is one of her favorite dishes, and she makes it a lot. We already had the bottle of wine."

"Do you have any of the food left over?"

"No, we ate it all except for some dregs that went down the disposal," said Bill. Then correcting himself, "No, that's not right. We still have almost all of the bean salad that we saved."

Acting like he was finished with this part of the examination, and without even touching his patients, the doctor struck a thoughtful pose and took a step back. Bill wondered if that was all he was going to do.

The doctor said a tech would be in to obtain blood for testing and that each would be given a specimen bottle to obtain a urine sample. He left, making no further comment.

As they waited for the technician to appear, Bill said, "A man of few words, I would say."

In ten minutes, the doctor returned. "I will get right down to the facts first and do some additional explaining later. While I was gone, I called the Centers for Disease Control in Atlanta and asked them to send a special treatment that will help you, if my suspicion about what you are both suffering from is correct. It will be here by this afternoon. I am treating you with a presumptive diagnosis of acute botulism poisoning contracted at your last meal thirty hours ago. If my diagnosis is correct, some of the botulinum toxin may still be circulating in your bloodstream. The antitoxin I have ordered will eliminate any poison still in your blood and not yet in your nerves. This treatment will shorten the duration and severity of your illness if it turns out to be botulism poisoning, which is what I think you have.

"You probably wonder why I am making this diagnosis without seeing any lab results and after looking at you briefly and asking only a few questions. You might also wonder how many patients I have treated with botulism poisoning. Full disclosure—that would be none, until now, if I am correct! I have read about the condition, especially with the rush of Botox now being used for cosmetic purposes. We have been on alert because of the remote possibility one of these treatments could result in an accidental overdose and require treatment for an affected person. Fortunately, we have not seen any, and honestly, I doubt we ever will.

"Now comes the catch-22. If we wait for a laboratory diagnosis, it is *always* too late for antitoxin and the disease is more serious with time. I should say that again. Not *usually*, *always*! The antitoxin is only effective up to thirty-six hours after the toxin enters the bloodstream. This means to provide the most effective treatment, you must accept a presumptive diagnosis every time using only circumstantial evidence. But there is a good part here. Antitoxin treatment given to a patient who does not have botulism poisoning results in no harm except for a rare allergic reaction, and that is entirely treatable. Now, it's your turn for questions." They had none.[2]

The doctor, in an official but still explanatory manner, said, "We will admit you to the neurology intensive care unit. This is not because you are desperately ill now, but because if we are correct and you have botulism poisoning, the disease could cause further problems with your nervous system, which could lead to difficulty breathing. We want you to be in a place where you can be observed closely and where equipment is available to assist you if necessary and without delay."

The couple was taken to an inpatient ward where they were placed in adjacent rooms. By two o'clock in the afternoon, both were receiving a slow intravenous drip of botulinum antitoxin. Bill was alert and curious. He asked the nurse about the antitoxin, where it came from and such. She said, "It came from the Centers for Disease Control in Atlanta and arrived by emergency courier. The staff there is on hand 24/7 and they promise to respond immediately."[3]

On the third day, results of their blood tests were returned. Everything was normal except . . . there was evidence of botulinum toxin type A in the blood of both. They were told it was the commonest and deadliest strain. The food from the restaurant had been tested earlier, and no toxin was found. The public health team, which had received their permission, had entered their apartment, obtained the bean salad for testing, and confirmed it contained botulinum toxin. Beans canned at the same time as those used for the salad prepared by Anne's mother also contained the toxin. All the remaining beans that had been canned were destroyed. Anne's mother had given all the salad to her daughter, a generous act that could have saved her own life.

The couple spent fourteen days in the hospital. They were mostly comfortable, but their stay was not without issues. Bill's double vision worsened before it gradually went away. He also had difficulty urinating and was catheterized several times before his waterworks got back on track. Anne's difficulty swallowing lasted about a week, and she was treated for constipation. Both received nasal oxygen, mostly as a precaution. The ventilator stood at the ready. Both dreaded it would be needed. It was not.

On the day of their discharge, the neurologist and infectious disease specialist who had been overseeing their care met with the couple to summarize the events of the last two weeks. They explained to Anne and Bill that they would be hearing things from them that they already knew, but they were doing this just to make sure that the two had been told everything they needed to know about what had happened to them. The neurologist and infectious disease specialist explained that the two must have ingested only a small amount of botulinum toxin at their meal on Saturday before they were admitted to the hospital. Tests of the ingredients at the restaurant where Bill got the carryout were found to be clear of any tainted food. This had been confirmed immediately. However, the bean salad remaining in their refrigerator tested positive for the toxin. The remaining jars of beans at Anne's mother's house tested negative but as a precaution, she disposed of the six remaining quarts, following the advice of the public health experts. It was agreed by all that the fact that the couple had eaten only a few bites of the salad might have saved their lives.

Anne and Bill were also told that being in bed for two weeks had the effect of taking the wind out of their sails. Both doctors assured the couple that two weeks from now, they would be back to their normal selves. This episode was a small hiccup in their lives, and they were lucky to have gotten through it with nothing more than what they had experienced.

Responding to an earlier question from Bill, the infectious disease specialist said, "Some of the concerning statistics you may have seen were from many years ago. Before 1950, between fifty and sixty percent of adults with botulism poisoning died, and infant botulism was not discovered until 1976. The incidence and mortality from the disease are much less now."

As the two specialists left the room, each was thinking to themselves, *That's the first one of these I have seen!*

Three days after seeing Anne and Bill in the emergency room, the doctor who first saw them learned about the lab results that confirmed his presumptive diagnosis of botulism poisoning. He realized he had not told Anne and Bill why he suspected botulism when he saw them. It was because of a story his uncle, a country doctor, had told him years ago. It went like this.

"I was called to see a family on a farm outside of the small town where I practiced. It was early in my practice, about 1959. On arrival, I saw a middle-aged farmer, his wife, and three children all in various degrees of distress with upset stomachs, vomiting, and weakness. All had been in good health prior to this episode, which started in the night and had gradually worsened during the day I saw them.

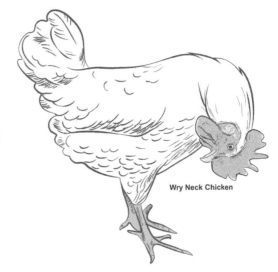

Descending paralysis from botulism poisoning in a chicken is apparent in the weakness of the neck muscles, causing a drooping of the head described as "wry neck."

Wry Neck Chicken

"The first thing that came to mind was food poisoning, although it didn't show the violent retching that usually results from that. The last meal they had eaten together the night before was homemade chili. Remembering what I had heard from a professor in medical school, I asked if they had chickens. When they said yes, I went into the barnyard, found the chickens, and noted several were walking around with a floppy, unsupported head and several others were dead. Knowing that farmers distributed unused table food to the livestock, I remembered my teacher's words and suspected the family and the chickens were suffering from the effects of eating the chili and that this could be a case of botulism poisoning.

"I didn't have much to offer them except to hold off eating for a day and call me tomorrow. Had this been a later time, they might have benefited from being in the hospital and receiving botulinum antitoxin, but it was not widely available then.

"The diagnosis was not confirmed, but homemade chili, five sick people, and wry-necked chickens told me I was seeing a family with botulism poisoning. The chickens had eaten the evidence, and it cost them their lives. The family survived, no thanks to me."[4]

6

World War II Sets the Stage

Botulinum toxin must be purified before it is deemed safe for human use. There was no pressing need for this process until the threat of the toxin being used as a biological weapon of war arose during World War II. To meet this threat, the United States had to uncover the secrets of the toxin.

Responding to pleas from British Prime Minister Winston Churchill, President Franklin D. Roosevelt launched a plan that included the establishment of a facility and the recruitment of a team of scientists to prepare for readiness in the event of biological warfare.[1] This effort unequivocally set the stage for the peaceful use of botulinum toxin in science and medicine. One man from this team of scientists would become the custodian of the toxin and would provide it to researchers for nearly four decades.

The next significant phase in the story of *Clostridium botulinum* toxin occurs in the middle of the twentieth century, when the world was on the brink of war for the second time in a generation. The United States joined the fray when Japan attacked Pearl Harbor on December 7, 1941. Within days, the Axis was formed when Germany and Italy, as allies of Japan, declared war on the United States. Based on prior acts by one of the belligerents, the Allied Forces—especially Britain—sought ways to defend against biological and chemical weapons like those employed in World War I.

England, the first of the Allies to get involved in World War II, was in a dark time. In the spring of 1940, Prime Minister Neville Chamberlain resigned seven months after Hitler's invasion of Poland, negating his earlier promise of "peace in our time." The country was ready for a change, and Britain's new prime minister, Winston Churchill, was ready for the challenge. After a decade of railing against Hitler's ambitions for the conquest of Europe, Churchill faced a monumental task. He approached it with zeal.

Sweeping westward across Europe, Hitler was employing a new mode of warfare. The combination of mobile infantry, supported by artillery and tanks, with close air cover overwhelmed all who faced it. This war machine carried out what was called *blitzkrieg* (lightning war). It had yet to meet the French, who had a superb army stationed behind the formidable Maginot Line. This series of fortifications on the border of France and Germany was thought to be impenetrable.

When the German attack skirted this defense by advancing through the French border with Belgium, it overwhelmed the French army. In days, the Germans were on the outskirts of Paris. The French—who the English thought would be a bulwark—surrendered in June, scarcely a month after Churchill took charge. This meant German bombers would be poised on French soil separated from the English mainland by the English Channel, a mere twenty-seven miles of water.

A priority for the new prime minister was to obtain help from the United States. Churchill was convinced that, despite the grit and tenacity of his own people, the war against Germany could not be won by England alone. His counterpart in the United States, President Roosevelt, was leading a country that was clawing its way out of the Great Depression. In the United States, there was little taste for another foreign war. The unrest troubling Europe, after what was touted "the war to end all wars," was something most Americans wanted no part in. Instead, many preferred a policy of isolation, as espoused by national hero Charles Lindbergh and other influential leaders.[2] A prevailing attitude was that the Atlantic Ocean was a buffer that (would have) allowed Americans to sit out the war while the Europeans dealt with their own problems. Furthermore, Roosevelt was anticipating a run for his third term, eschewing a precedent set by George Washington. (After Roosevelt's election for a fourth term in 1944, the Twenty-Second Amendment to the Constitution was passed in 1951, limiting the presidential term of office to two terms.)

Though involvement in Europe's affairs was unpopular with many, the president realized America must come to the aid of England for that country to withstand the German onslaught. Moreover, a loss by the English would negatively affect the United States, whether we joined the war or remained on the sideline. To President Roosevelt—or FDR, as the president was called—letting that nation fall while we did nothing to help would be unconscionable. Facing this dilemma, FDR saw the need for a firsthand assessment of conditions in Britain.

To learn more about the state of his beleaguered ally, FDR tapped William Donovan for the job. Donovan had served as a United States attorney for the Western District of New York and later as assistant attorney general in the Coolidge administration before establishing a successful law practice on Wall Street. Donovan also happened to be the most decorated American soldier in World War I. He earned the four highest military awards: the Medal of Honor, the Distinguished Service Cross, two Distinguished Service Medals, and the Silver Star, as well as three Purple Hearts. The president's instructions for Donovan were to assess the situation in Britain and in his judgment determine how likely it was for this country to prevail.[3]

During two trips to England, in July and December 1940, Donovan met with Churchill and King George VI. Donovan was shown the new Spitfire fighter planes, the novel radar-warning system, and other secret coastal-defense facilities. And, perhaps most important, he was introduced to the need to gather information about the enemy and use it in propaganda and subversion. It was a fateful visit. Churchill, for the sake of England, understood the importance of Donovan's mission and sought to use it to persuade his visitor that the United States should join England in the war effort.

No immediate action was taken by FDR after Donovan's return. The dire warning his envoy conveyed did put FDR on notice though. The president knew he should act, but only after the country was ready for the news. Among the topics that came out of Donovan's report was Britain's urgent need to replenish their depleted navy. There would be no help from the French, who had destroyed the heart of their fleet when they scuttled seventy-seven ships in the Toulon Harbor. This drastic measure was the only way to keep the ships out of the hands of the German invaders.

As an island nation, England believed having a strong navy was essential for their defense. The situation for Britain was dire, and FDR recognized the urgency. He agreed to send fifty aged destroyers to Churchill in September 1940. All the ships had been scheduled for decommissioning, so there was no strategic loss for the United States. To help influence public opinion, Roosevelt knew it was necessary to receive something from Britain in return, and an agreement was struck.[4]

On delivery of the ships, the United States was compensated with a ninety-nine-year lease for bases in Bermuda and several other British ports in the Caribbean. The price paid by the administration was the risk of alienating voters who wanted their country to avoid war at any cost. The strategic advantage achieved with the new bases took some of the sting out of the deal with those voters.

The Intelligence Services

Events in Europe, and the sobering information received from Donovan, convinced FDR to make a bold move. Over objections from some in the military and from the head of the FBI, J. Edgar Hoover, FDR established the Office of Coordination of Information (COI) in July 1941 with William Donovan as its head.[5] This was an intelligence operation established loosely on the model of the agencies Donovan had observed in England. As conditions in Europe steadily deteriorated, options for the United States gradually narrowed. The sudden and unprovoked attack by the Japanese changed everything. Four days later, Germany, along with Italy, declared war on the United States. World War II was underway, and the president, operating on a war footing, was met with no objections from the people as he formed a strategy to meet the challenges he faced.

Dirty Tricks

While waging war on two fronts—including North Africa and the vast Pacific Ocean and islands—in June 1942, FDR disbanded the COI and by executive order formed the Office of Strategic Services (OSS), an operation that was more proactive in dealing with the exigencies of war. FDR again tapped William Donovan to be its head. The role of the OSS was to obtain information and carry out sabotage. The OSS engaged in shadow operations while striving to thwart all manner of hostile ambitions from enemy nations during World War II.

The timely development of ways to deter threats from the enemy, including chemical warfare as used in World War I and even biological warfare, was a high priority for Donovan. He had been introduced to these strategies while in England and saw the need for them in his own country.[6] The OSS director, who had started as a colonel in the army, later rose to major general and would head the premier US intelligence organization that would operate on all fronts as it aided the war effort at home and worldwide.

OSS agents fought a covert war, replete with daring and adventure. Those recruited included a movie actor, Sterling Hayden; a baseball player polyglot, Mo Berg, a catcher who played fifteen seasons in the major leagues; famous chef Julia Child and her husband, Paul, a diplomat; John Ford, a noted movie director; and others. Less celebrated but useful recruits were psychiatrists, gunsmiths, engineers, chemists, policemen, detectives, prisoners, safecrackers, bankers, journalists, and gangsters. Also included were former war prisoners and refugees.

The military assumed some tasks of the now-defunct COI while also working with Donovan's team at the OSS. The OSS moved ahead in development, seeking new friends and along the way acquiring the inevitable new enemies. A unique feature of the new organization was the inclusion of civilians working alongside the military. Another special feature was nearly a quarter of the team were women.[7]

William "Wild Bill" Donovan was a man who would cut corners when it was necessary to get things done. He both cooperated and competed with the Armed Forces (more the latter, from their perspective). J. Edgar Hoover hated Donovan, a feeling that Donovan returned.

Until President Truman disbanded the OSS in 1945, some of its secret projects included the development of methods—sometimes bizarre—to sow mischief, hamper enemy efforts, and devise ways to counteract threats. Some of those activities included the study, but not the actual deployment, of lethal toxins, along with other methods that could be used on both offense and defense. In just two years, those activities were continued by the Central Intelligence Agency, after it was formed in 1947 to replace the OSS and headed by Porter J. Goss. The goal of this agency contrasted starkly with the selfless efforts of a unique group of young men assigned to projects in the realm of pure science that would achieve a far-reaching positive effect.

This type of highly secret research, launched after the attack on Pearl Harbor, took place at a new army facility in 1943 at Camp Detrick (previously named Detrick Field) in Frederick, Maryland. The government later renamed the facility Fort Detrick, and it became the headquarters for pioneering militarily relevant research that continues today, including far-reaching biomedical research and development. More than two dozen scientists staffed the initial core facility that later expanded. The initial group ranged from young scientists in training to recent graduates who were only beginning their career. Many were in their twenties, and someone who had reached thirty was considered an old man.

7

Camp Detrick—US Army Biological Warfare Laboratories

Now into the second year of World War II, the United States is battling on two fronts as the nation fights for its survival.

In 1943, the United States was battling fiercely against the combined forces of Germany, Italy, and Japan. The country faced an uncertain future as it played catch-up after a slow start. Elsewhere, the German aerial bombing campaign over England, which had begun in September 1940, continued unabated until May 1941. In these raids, bombs and incendiaries destroyed property and dealt death to the civilian population. These weapons were conventional: they demolished buildings, spawned raging fires, and caused civilian casualties. The home guard used the tools at hand, wielded by crews with shovels and fire hoses, for destroyed property and litters and ambulances for the civilian dead and injured. What was happening now was bad enough, but even more harrowing images wracked the minds of British leaders. They fretted about what would come next. So far, their country had not been hit with the "other thing"—that is, the Germans had not resorted to chemical or biological warfare. But how long would it be before they did?[1]

The British were hard-pressed but did not break. From the continent, the Germans launched pilotless buzz bombs that rained down on England. These rockets could be equipped to deliver a variety of biological weapons with devastating effect. The enemy had used alternative weapons in warfare during World War I. Would they do it again? This was not a question that could remain unanswered for long.[2]

(Information available only later revealed that Hitler did not plan to use biological warfare because he was afraid the Allies would fight back the same way.)

THE PRESIDENT ACTS

Once President Roosevelt established a novel biological warfare effort at Camp Detrick, events moved ahead rapidly. While speed was a priority, secrecy was tantamount. News of the camp and its mission were restricted to an inner circle of responsible individuals. George W. Merck, head of a prominent pharmaceutical firm that still bears his name, had the job of overseeing all aspects of this effort.[3] While this was being accomplished, the secrecy surrounding Camp Detrick and the task assigned was said to be matched by only one other war-related program: the ultra-secret Manhattan Project that was charged with creating a nuclear chain reaction and finding a way to weaponize it. The first goal in this task was achieved in 1942.[4] It took place at the University of Chicago in a squash court located under the stands of a football stadium named after the venerable coach Amos Alonso Stagg. The chain reaction technology was soon employed to build the first atomic bomb at Oak Ridge, Tennessee.

ESTABLISHMENT OF THE BIOLOGICAL WARFARE CENTER

With World War II underway and no time to waste, the US military's scientific effort dealing with biological warfare started work at Camp Detrick, Maryland, in 1943. Camp Detrick was renamed Fort Detrick in 1956 and continues to hold this name.

The monumental accomplishments there—especially during the critical early years—focused on key issues related to the war effort. Initially, an unlikely group of scientists assembled in an improbable environment: a makeshift facility little more than a tar-paper shack. It was named the "Black Maria," after the building Thomas Edison constructed in 1892 to be the first moving picture studio. The group achieved amazing results as they unlocked secrets vital to the war effort and beyond.

In the beginning, the group's charge was to study certain biological agents capable of being weaponized. This effort combined a sense of urgency with the need for secrecy. One of the tasks was to assess the possibility of the enemy using the most lethal of biological toxins, *Clostridium botulinum*. They needed to find out how this substance acted, how it could be dispersed, and the best way to mount a defense if it was used. There was concern on the part of the British that this toxin could be employed to poison the reservoirs that supplied drinking water.

The biological warfare facility of the US Army sprang up on the site of Detrick Field, a small airport only fifty-five miles from Washington, DC. Initially it was a site for selected, though not clearly defined, activities shrouded in secrecy and with oversight by the OSS.[5] Detrick Field consisted of little more than a grass airstrip that had been used as an emergency landing site and for limited military purposes. The only buildings that remained were empty barracks and an unused hangar. The runways were usable and an abandoned control tower still stood. What became of Detrick Field, a remote spot until its metamorphosis into Camp Detrick, was an example of hiding in plain sight. In addition to its proximity to the capital, the facility was only a few miles from Catoctin Mountain, the site of the presidential retreat Shangri-La that was renamed Camp David by President Eisenhower.

The first scientific laboratory, clad in tar paper secured by battens and newly constructed on the site, the "Black Maria,"[6] was the center for top-secret research efforts, including the unlocking of secrets about botulinum toxin. Scientists were said to have worked in the laboratory with loaded .45-caliber pistols and lived in barracks within the restricted military environment of Camp Detrick.[7] The equipment installation was closely supervised by the scientists who were delving into the secrets of death-dealing poisons. Heading up the project was Dr. Ira Baldwin from the University of Wisconsin. He was selected for the job partly because of his belief: "The problem is simple. If you can do it with a test tube, you can do it with a 10,000-gallon tank with equal safety and perhaps more."

This can-do attitude held more power at the time because the question of whether the enemy would use biological warfare remained unanswered. Churchill, for one, was clambering for help. "He should know" was a prevailing attitude. This caused leaders in the US government to take actions so the country would be as ready as possible, even at the risk of overpreparing. This was the situation faced as events at Camp Detrick took shape.

Botulinum Toxin in 1943

A significant body of knowledge about *Clostridium botulinum* had been compiled in the 121 years since Justinus Kerner's original work. This was useful, but there was more to be learned. The young scientists working at Camp Detrick during World War II knew this much about one of the deadly substances they would be working with:

- *Clostridium botulinum* produces an exotoxin that is lethal in minuscule amounts.
- Epidemics of botulism poisoning in the United States from tainted olives appeared twenty years before. A study of these events provided valuable new information about the toxin's behavior. Now, largely thanks to stringent rules applied to the food processing industry (canning), botulism was a rare sporadic and mostly foodborne event.
- Botulism poisoning first affects the autonomic nervous system and later nervous connection of voluntary muscles, including in the limbs. It starts with weakness beginning at the top (eyes and lids) and descending through the throat reaches the muscles governing breathing, resulting in death to half of those affected.
- In 1926, Dr. Hermann Sommer of the George Williams Hooper Foundation at the University of California, San Francisco, produced a crude form of botulinum toxin capable of inducing paralysis in laboratory animals.
- There is no known cure for botulism poisoning.
- Use of botulinum toxin in warfare is possible in theory, but questions about practicality remain.

A task assigned to these scientists included the study of deadly toxins. Their efforts concentrated on two: *Clostridium botulinum* and shellfish toxin (saxitoxin). These were of special interest to the directors of the laboratory. Although a great deal was known about the clinical characteristics of botulism poisoning and the bacteria, *Clostridium botulinum*, the toxin it produced had not been fully described in a purified form. In addition, its precise effect on the nervous system and how to counteract it was unknown.

By 1945, and the end of World War II that celebrated an Allied victory, a new phase began in the history of the deadly *Clostridium botulinum* toxin. Before peace was reached, in just a few months of whirlwind activity, scientists at Camp Detrick succeeded in purifying the crystalline toxin for the first time. They were also successful in providing an explanation of how the toxin affected the nervous system. With this knowledge gained, they created a toxoid capable of producing a vaccine to protect against this molecule and set the stage for development of an antitoxin for treatment. Moreover, the confluence of information assembled in the laboratory and from other sources at Camp Detrick led to a firm belief that botulinum toxin was not likely to be employed as an offensive weapon.

There were several unlikely stars in this lineup of fledgling scientists. Twenty-seven-year-old biochemist Carl Lamanna led a small group that was the first to purify botulinum toxin type A, which would become Botox a half century later.[8] Twenty-three-year-old surgery resident Arthur

Guyton, drafted from his position at Massachusetts General Hospital in Boston, carried out brilliant research showing how the toxin affected nerve action on muscles.[9] This information was key as indications for botulinum toxin treatment expanded. Thirty-three-year-old Edward Schantz, the "old man," kept this toxin culture alive while he supplied dozens of basic scientists with toxin for their experiments. Best known of these scientists receiving toxin was Alan Scott, who for thirty years worked to develop a drug from botulinum toxin type A and named it Oculinum, which we now know as Botox.

Work carried out in the laboratory slowed with the end of World War II. The young scientists who had been originally drafted or enlisted to support the war effort shifted their work to pursue scientific endeavors in civilian life. That did not end the activity at Camp Detrick; instead, it changed the focus.

The wartime deeds by the team at Camp Detrick continue to influence our lives today. On the positive side, this is largely because of one man who stayed behind, Dr. Edward Schantz. He remained in the laboratory, first in the military and later as a civilian, until he retired in 1971.[10] Remaining at Fort Detrick, Dr. Schantz continued to monitor the toxins left over from the war effort. He provided small amounts of saxitoxin to food scientists who conducted assays testing shellfish to ensure they were free of toxin and safe for consumption. Dealing with poisons remaining at Fort Detrick, Schantz's most consequential work was the production and optimization of cultures of botulinum toxin type A. For decades, he supplied this material free for use in the laboratory and supported the work of more than 150 qualified scientists worldwide.[11]

When Ed Schantz left Fort Detrick in 1971, he shifted the botulinum toxin culture program to his new laboratory at the University of Wisconsin-Madison. The 1970 executive order to destroy all toxins held by the CIA that could be used for warfare carried the exception that "small amounts" that could be useful for health purposes could be spared. Criteria and authority for decisions dealing with these toxins were not spelled out. Edward Schantz, it seems, decided on his own to continue dealing with the toxin as he had been doing.

In 1972, retired from Fort Detrick and at the Wisconsin Food Research Institute, Schantz agreed to provide Alan Scott with botulinum toxin type A for his first primate experiments. This began a twenty-year collaboration, leading to the first botulinum toxin injection in a human in 1978.

Around the middle of the twentieth century, discoveries related to botulinum toxin advances in basic science and medicine may have depended more on the actions of the scientist responding to a prevailing sense of urgency than on a litany of rules and regulations imposed by others. Think of those researchers charting their own course as they created the atomic bomb. Were their actions pursued properly and ethically? Were shortcuts taken? Was the work done for the betterment of humankind?

There is room for argument on each point. Guided by their own genius and responding to a plea from the government that was acting on behalf of the people, the scientists guiding the Manhattan Project accepted a challenge, did what they believed was right, and delivered a product that ended World War II. One can suspect most of the rules they followed were self-imposed; they were not alone in working this way. This could have been a prevailing attitude throughout much of the scientific community, including in the lab at Camp Detrick.

Today, a cynic may believe rules are fair game and they are only to be broken, or worked around, if you can get away with it. In this scenario, rules can replace ethical practice as the person's guiding factor, sparing the doer from any personal responsibility. Retroactively judging the behavior of researchers, beginning in the war years and continuing through the 1950s and 1960s, requires a unique filter. With fewer rules back then, decisions were made based on ethics and a willingness to take personal responsibility to do the right thing. Behavior was not dictated; it was chosen. Many of the current regulations are likely to have little effect on those ethical researchers or medical practitioners committed to doing the right thing on their own. A belief of some may be that arbitrary rules only slow progress for those who are bound to employ their own good judgment and do the right thing. The ones who need to be bridled by these rules, some believe, are probably those few whose dubious goal is to find a way to get around them—to cheat.

There is no way to prove it, but it is possible that the work accomplished by Alan Scott in developing botulinum toxin type A for medical use (and who knows how much good work by others at the time) may never have been completed if every rule in effect today—some might call it red tape—had been strictly followed. This also could have been the case when a small group of young scientists at Camp Detrick first purified the toxin, and one member of the group kept it alive and made it available for half a century!

For us today, this is only speculation. Creating the purified toxin was important, and it eventually proved a benefit to humankind. But equally important was the good judgment that prevailed in Edward Schantz when he circumvented an arbitrary rule, thereby allowing a useful drug to be developed from a deadly toxin.

Before the health-promoting effects of botulinum toxin type A were achieved with material supplied by Ed Schantz and used by Alan Scott in his laboratory and clinic, a dark side of toxins from Fort Detrick was exposed. CIA agents pursuing shrouded projects planned clandestine operations using these toxins to plan assassinations and support assisted suicides. And there was more. Lysergic acid obtained from a reputable manufacturer was being tested as a possible truth serum in experiments that included surreptitious poisoning of an agent that ended in tragedy. The details were shared in a book by Stephen Kinzer titled *Poisoner in Chief: Sidney Gottlieb and the CIA Search for Mind Control.*

8

Fort Detrick and the CIA

The facility at Camp Detrick had assumed a Jekyll-and-Hyde personality.

It started with a young man from New York. He had a limp from a club foot and a slight speech impediment. He was searching for a school that offered course material in agricultural biology. That was the educational path Sidney Gottlieb wanted to pursue. He sought the advice of Dr. Ira Baldwin, assistant dean of the College of Agriculture at the University of Wisconsin. Baldwin said it was necessary for Gottlieb to first take preliminary coursework at another institution if he hoped to gain a position at Wisconsin. Gottlieb enrolled at the University of Arkansas to complete the requisite coursework and then went to Wisconsin, where he was guided by Dr. Baldwin. Gottlieb graduated in 1940 with honors, and three years later, having been encouraged by the dean, he received his doctorate in biochemistry from the California Institute of Technology.[1]

Young Dr. Gottlieb was unable to take an active part in the war effort because of his physical status. He had thought it would not hamper him, but he was wrong. After working at several jobs, including with the Food and Drug Administration and the National Research Council, he landed a position as a research associate at the University of Maryland and began to study fungi. With his wife's encouragement and sensing the needs of a growing family, Sidney moved them to a primitive cabin twenty miles from Washington, DC. There he enjoyed a bucolic existence, at least outside of work. His time at home with his family was fulfilling; but at his job, the scientist believed he was mired in a midlevel position. Though happy with gardening, milking goats, and pitching in with other chores as he settled into a comfortable family life, Sidney Gottlieb sought more.[2]

By 1943, Dr. Ira Baldwin had assumed his role as scientific director of the United States Army Biological Warfare Laboratories at Camp Detrick. This facility became a key component of the nation's biological warfare service. Government authorities promised Baldwin he would receive whatever he wanted unless the Manhattan Project asked first. The new director was instrumental in selecting the site at Detrick Field, which was promptly renamed Camp Detrick. After this, he assembled a staff that grew to more than a thousand. The man Baldwin had mentored at Wisconsin, Sidney Gottlieb, was too young to serve under his former professor at the beginning. But later, the facility played a significant role in Gottlieb's career. In a strange turn of fate, he, in turn, would act in a way that cast aspersions on the reputation of Fort Detrick through his efforts as a special, though unusual, agent with the CIA.

Sidney Gottlieb joined the CIA in 1951 and was immediately assigned to a three-month course aimed at teaching him how to become an effective spy. After this, his job was to create a band of agents, including biochemists, who would apply their skills pursuing offbeat tasks for the organization. This work was mostly related to thought control, including the use of chemical agents. It led to what was called the Bluebird Project. The meaning of this appellation applied to the aim of the activity, which was to find ways to make people reveal information. They would "sing like a bird." In this era of so-called brainwashing, which was deeply beset with concerns of leaked secrets and high-level spying, the effort seemed important. Success of the project would be measured by how much information could be uncovered using the skills developed, as well as how effectively this kind of activity could be defended against.[3]

One of Gottlieb's most energetic pursuits was the study of lysergic acid (LSD), including finding a reliable source. Sandoz, a pharmaceutical company in Switzerland, was becoming disenchanted with the product and wanted out. Back home in the United States, a domestic pharmaceutical company established a new process for manufacturing LSD, which meant that the drug could now be mass-produced. The CIA agent who reported this development to his superiors noted that the government had access to a home-based supply of LSD by the "ton." The company kept details of the full process confidential and made up a special batch of LSD for the CIA. They were able to produce the drug in volume and agreed to supply it to the CIA. This resulted in an order for $400,000 worth of the chemical. It turned out to be the largest subcontract ever carried out by the CIA.[4]

Since the 1960s, LSD has been listed as illegal and is a Schedule I substance under the Controlled Substances Act. It joined heroin in this class of drugs, which has a high potential for abuse while serving no legitimate medical purpose.[5] LSD had arrived in the United States in 1949 and was originally perceived as a psychomimetic capable of producing a model psychosis. But by the mid nineteen fifties, intellectuals in Southern California redefined LSD as a psychedelic capable of producing a psychical effect.[6]

An example of how Sidney Gottlieb was operating at the time is demonstrated by an act he carried out in 1953. He invited a group of CIA colleagues to a retreat and then, unbeknownst to them, spiked their after-dinner drinks with LSD. His aim was to observe the behavior of those who ingested the potion and use what he learned to find better ways to employ the drug for what was loosely described as "mind control." Frank Olson, a CIA officer guest based out of the Special Operations Division at Camp Detrick, was one of those who received a drink spiked with LSD. He suffered a profound mind-altering effect and was not able to rebound to his normal state after being given the drug. After a week, when Olson continued to behave in a seriously disturbed and bizarre manner, Gottlieb decided something needed to be done. With no letup in his symptoms, Olson was sent to New York to be seen by a doctor for a special examination. Another agent accompanied Olson. There the drugged agent was seen by Dr. Greenberg, a physician under contract to the CIA and specializing in the effects of mind-control drugs.

Nothing conclusive was said to have been determined at the appointment. Then, back in the hotel, Olson left his bed at 2:30 a.m. and jumped or was thrown out of the window of his room on the thirteenth floor of the Statler (later Pennsylvania) Hotel across the street from Penn Station. His death was called a suicide in a rush to close the case, and it remained so for more than a decade until the family had the body exhumed and reexamined. The authorities then changed the cause of death to "cause unknown pending police investigation." Mrs. Olson and her family remained convinced the agent was murdered for fear he would reveal secrets the CIA wanted to be kept. Finally, President Gerald Ford invited the family to the Oval Office, where he offered an official apology. The family received a

$750,000 settlement from the government in 1976.[7] A later civil suit was dismissed.[8]

Poisoner in Chief paints a dark role for Camp Detrick, later named Fort Detrick, during the 1950s and 1960s, and Sidney Gottlieb's role is key. Stephen Kinzer, the author, describes Gottlieb's use of two deadly toxins created and held exclusively at Camp Detrick. They were not his own, but the CIA Special Operations Department (SOD) stationed at the facility had access and made them available through connections that were never fully disclosed.[9] Later, when asked under oath at a Senate hearing, Edward Schantz said, "I didn't know it at the time."

One of the biological poisons, botulinum toxin type A, eventually obtained by Gottlieb, was purified for the first time at Camp Detrick and used to create a vaccine to protect troops on D-Day and a toxoid to produce an equine antitoxin. Another lethal toxin that was harvested at the same time from shellfish was collected and purified at Camp Detrick for potential but at the time unstated use by the government. Ed Schantz retained supplies of both. Schantz provided small consignments of toxin to qualified researchers and food scientists for specific and accountable reasons, such as physiology experiments or food assays. Most of the core group of young scientists assembled during the war years had been drafted or had volunteered for duty. After their time at Camp Detrick, they went on to serve society while pursuing long and fruitful careers. But there were others who may unwittingly have worked more closely with the CIA, as was apparently the case with Schantz.

New Employment for Deadly Toxins

In April 1960, a special plane employed in secrecy by the CIA and United States Air Force took off from a base in Peshawar, Pakistan. It carried the pilot, Captain Francis Gary Powers, to 70,000 feet. This altitude was attained to put the plane beyond the reach of those on the ground while cameras in the plane photographed military installations and other places of strategic interest in Russia. Captain Powers was conducting a special CIA mission. These U-2 flights were kept as highly sensitive secrets, and each mission had to be personally approved by President Eisenhower.

Approval for this mission was denied at first. The reason was the president would be meeting with the Soviet leader Nikita Khrushchev barely a week after the flight was scheduled. Eisenhower did not want there to be any possibility of his needing to explain if the flight was discovered. Later, after the CIA convinced Eisenhower that there was no possibility of trouble with the mission, he relented. As a result of the disastrous events occurring later, Eisenhower was forced to deal with the most humiliating experience of his presidency. He had to admit that he had lied to Khrushchev. With this, the summit that had been scheduled immediately after the meeting in Paris was canceled.[10]

The U-2 pilots were supplied with a suicide option for use if they were captured and threatened with torture. The device at the time contained cyanide in a glass ampoule, but concerns about the possibility of accidental employment led to a search for another option. The CIA needed to devise a new method for suicide to be used by these daring pilots, if they chose that course. The CIA's response might have been the capstone of Sidney Gottlieb's career in designing devices.

Francis Gary Powers was given a silver dollar to be worn around his neck as a medallion. The coin's bottom edge had a hole, through which a hollow pin was inserted. This hollow pin acted as a sheath for a thinner pin with grooves along the side and near the tip. The purpose of this device was to offer the option of painless suicide. To activate the device, the sheath could be removed from the silver dollar and the inner pin pulled out to reveal a sticky brown material in fine grooves along the shaft and at the tip. The grooves held shellfish toxin (saxitoxin). Scratching the skin with the poison-laden pin enabled a lethal dose of the poison, measured in micrograms, to enter the system. The result of this act would be near-instantaneous death. The toxin was a product of Fort Detrick, and the design was the work of Sidney Gottlieb.[11]

Gary Powers took off in his U-2 plane just before the president was to go to Paris for the international summit. Flying at more than thirteen miles above the ground, an altitude thought to render his plane undetectable, Powers' plane was hit by an explosive device from an advanced-design Soviet rocket. The rocket ripped off both the plane's extra-long wings. Immediately the fuselage pointed upward, and the plane began to fall backward. In the rush, Powers was not able to activate the switch to destroy the plane before he ejected. As he floated down in his parachute, the pilot was aware of his options and decided to hit the ground and face being captured.

Powers survived the fall, and his captors took his "suicide silver dollar" and carried out a detailed analysis. Although they confirmed the sticky brown substance was lethal, they did not identify it as saxitoxin or uncover its origin at Fort Detrick. Powers was tried, convicted of espionage, and was sentenced to eleven years in a Soviet prison. After serving two years, he was released in 1962, in exchange for the Soviet spy Rudolf Abel.[12]

When he first returned to the United States, Powers was met with derision. But as emotions surrounding the event cooled, he was hailed as a hero and given a medal for his service. After he died in 1977, Powers was presented posthumously with the Silver Star for gallantry in action. (More than six decades later, improved U-2 aircraft are still in service and provide unique benefits in what are described as "lightly contested areas."[13])

Only five suicide silver dollars were fabricated, and one is on display at the International Spy Museum in Washington, DC. These suicide kits were intended for each pilot, or "driver" as they were called. None were used. However, the word *saxitoxin* must have become known to many in Washington because this was the only toxin held by the CIA at Fort Detrick that was discussed extensively during the 1975 Church Committee hearings.

Another of Gottlieb's innovations for assassination involved botulinum toxin type A. The target for assassination was Patrice Lumumba, a Congolese politician who served as the first prime minister of the Republic of the Congo. Desperate for economic support, Lumumba sought help from the Soviets, who were eager to take advantage of this mineral-rich country. Not only were the Americans concerned but also were the Belgians, who had originally colonized this part of Africa.

The CIA man, with the help of the SOD team at Fort Detrick, designed a kit to include a vial of liquefied botulinum toxin type A. It was diluted but retained a lethal concentration. Also included were a syringe and needle, rubber gloves, a face mask for safety, and a bottle of chlorine to deactivate the toxin if that became necessary. Gottlieb personally delivered this to the CIA operative in Léopoldville. He gave the man, who was the section chief, instructions to put the toxin in anything that the intended victim would be likely to put into his mouth, like food or toothpaste. The section chief was not enthusiastic about carrying out the plan. After Gottlieb left, the kit was stored in a safe. Nobody could be found who had both access to Lumumba and a willingness to deliver the toxin. Subsequent events occurring within months of Gottlieb's visit eliminated the need for action, and the toxin remained out of harm's way in the safe. It was finally destroyed after Lumumba was captured and eventually killed by a firing squad.[14]

Later a CIA plot to assassinate Fidel Castro included a plan to put botulinum toxin type A on fifty cigars and present the box as a gift to the Cuban leader. The cigars were Cohiba, Castro's favorite brand. It would be a laborious job to unwrap, dose with the toxin, and rewrap so many cigars. As with other plans to assassinate or otherwise disable Castro, this plot was never carried out because of the strict security that surrounded the leader.[15]

In his testimony before the Church Committee in 1975, Dr. Edward Schantz, the only witness to testify on the third day, was asked if he knew of the CIA connection at Fort Detrick. His answer was: "I didn't know at the time." This was immediately qualified by his statement, "But I wouldn't have been surprised."[16]

9

The Government Steps In

A Senate committee investigates the CIA response to an executive order and expresses concerns about activities involving poisons and toxins carried out at Fort Detrick.

Amid rumors of abusive practices by the CIA and in response to an international treaty, President Richard Nixon issued an executive order in 1970. It declared that the United States would abandon "offensive preparations for and the use of toxins as a method of warfare."[1] This order included exemptions for agents that could be used for peaceful purposes and that could be retained in what were described as "small amounts." Not strictly defined, "small amount" could mean three teaspoonfuls—enough to kill the entire population of the world if it were pure botulinum toxin. A literal interpretation of the order meant that *all* existing American toxin stocks would be destroyed unless there was a good reason to not do so. But this left unanswered who was authorized to determine what was a small amount, what was useful, and what was peaceful.

Compliance with the order to destroy all poisons and toxins remaining at Fort Detrick would have included destruction of the botulinum toxin. This did not happen. Remember, twenty-five years earlier, shortly after the end of World War II, Edward Schantz had become the de facto custodian of all the poisons at Fort Detrick. As such he considered it in his purview to supply small amounts of these materials to support the legitimate work of responsible scientists.

Under his watchful eye, Dr. Schantz saw botulinum toxin becoming a vital tool in the laboratory. Though it was a deadly poison, the toxin became just another useful tool for researchers when employed properly. When

Schantz left Fort Detrick, the ban on toxins notwithstanding, he continued to act as he had: dealing with botulinum toxin on his own terms. Later events revealed that he acted wisely and in the best interests of the scientific community and those it served. When Dr. Edward Schantz joined the University of Wisconsin-Madison in 1971, he brought with him an abundance of competence, including the skill to create and maintain a culture of botulinum toxin.

Shortly after his move to Wisconsin, Schantz began to supply Doctor Alan Scott with the toxin in a collaboration that lasted twenty years. Instead of the story of Clostridium botulinum ending with an executive order, Schantz's decision made possible the eventual development of Botox. However, it was not until a Senate Committee hearing in 1975 that botulinum A toxin was recognized as one of the poisons and given retroactive exemption from destruction and the panel of senators authorized Ed Schantz as its custodian. The senators recognized the value of this material for the study of the causes of human illness and its vital role in finding better ways to treat disease. The committee's decision was to allow Dr. Edward Schantz to continue to use the toxins according to his best judgment. He remained as the custodian of materials in his possession without naming them specifically.

Working in his own laboratory in Wisconsin, Schantz continued to manage the botulinum culture as he had been but now in support of a new and exciting research effort. The work required to satisfy Alan Scott's needs for the toxin became more demanding with the onset of clinical trials that eventually required thousands of doses administered by two hundred investigators. The botulinum toxin culture used for the first human trials was the same used earlier in the initial primate studies. Replacing the old, a new culture provided toxin to Scott shortly after his first injection of a human. It was known as 79-11. (Toxin batches were named for the year and month they were prepared; 79-11 means November 1979.) This hardy culture lasted for more than fifteen years and supplied all of the clinical trials. During this period, the toxin's quality was assured by regular assays carried out by Schantz and his associate at Wisconsin, Dr. Eric Johnson. This batch of toxin lasted until its replacement was prepared by Allergan and was approved by the FDA in 1997, six years after they purchased Oculinum Inc. from Alan Scott.[2]

THE CIA AT FORT DETRICK

It was well known in government circles that activities at Fort Detrick were shrouded in secrecy. In many cases, records were scant, if kept at all, and those making decisions were in the shadows and not always held accountable. The Special Operations Division of the CIA, which was said to have destroyed records in the 1960s, dealt closely with selected personnel at Fort Detrick while they maintained a presence at the facility. The president's executive order to destroy toxins and poisons held by the CIA had not been carried out, and rumors of misuse of the toxins were afloat. It was time to investigate these actions. A Select Senate Oversight Committee would do it.

The Senate hearings were held in September 1975. Senator Frank Church, who had been an officer in the US Army Intelligence Corps, was the committee's chairman. He opened the hearing by saying: "[These hearings are] . . . serious business . . . the CIA has been involved in assassination plots. . . . These plots involved planned attempts on the heads of state of two countries and would employ poisons produced and possibly held at Fort Detrick." The chairman explained these hearings would be "an inquiry into a case in which direct orders of the President of the United States were evidently disobeyed by employees of the CIA."[3]

The purpose of the hearings was to "illuminate" the need to make certain in the future that federal law enforcement and intelligence agencies performed their duties in ways that did not infringe on the rights of American citizens. It was acknowledged that government agencies had done bad things. The country would benefit from disclosure of these wrongdoings and establish policies that would keep them from happening in the future. In the process, the government would do its best to put right any wrongs that were done.

On the first two days, the testimony was mainly from William Colby, the CIA director, and Richard Helms, a high-ranking CIA officer.[4] They admitted that assassination attempts had been planned by others in the CIA and that a suicide device to replace a cyanide ampoule had been designed but the suicide devices were never used, and the assassination attempts were not carried out. During this testimony, both saxitoxin and botulinum toxin were mentioned but nothing was decided. Two days of inconclusive testimony ended with a promise that more would be learned about the Fort Detrick toxins on the final day of the hearings, when the only witness would be Dr. Edward Schantz.[5]

What effect would these hearings have on Schantz, who had spent the prime of his career, twenty-eight years, at Fort Detrick, before retiring four years earlier?

World War II was behind. America was embroiled in a new kind of war, the Cold War, and once again Fort Detrick and its dealings with the CIA were in the limelight. As early as 1958, the US Senate's concern about actions by the CIA that could have led to the supervision of this organization by the Senate was discussed, but there was no resolution. These issues were not new. The lawmakers decided it was time to learn more so they could deal with the CIA appropriately.

The first two days of testimony dealt with the CIA's involvement in the development of biological warfare materials at the army's biological laboratory at Fort Detrick. The committee wanted to know the whereabouts of the shellfish toxin produced at the fort and about the CIA's use of other chemicals and drugs. Most of these questions were for Director William Colby and Richard Helms, but several other officers and operatives working for the CIA were quizzed. On the third day, the committee heard the testimony of Dr. Edward Schantz.

Testimony in the first two days revealed the CIA had been seeking a replacement for the current cyanide delivery system for suicide by agents in case of capture. Such an ampoule was issued to agents in special cases during World War II, but there was concern the method currently being deployed could be prone to accidents. This led to the CIA seeking a more reliable device using equally lethal shellfish toxin available at Fort Detrick. This testimony disclosed that the new suicide kit containing Fort Detrick shellfish toxin was poised for use in a U-2 flight by Gary Powers. In other plots, botulinum toxin was selected to be the agent to kill Patrice Lumumba and Fidel Castro. Neither action was carried out.

Were these projects justified? Even if they were never carried out, did the intent render them subject to penalty? Did the acts of the intended victims justify what was being proposed? Do the heat of war and the laudable intention of the planner change the rules? These are hard questions, and the answers may never be found. Though unpleasant to consider, questions like these will continue to be posed and answers will be elusive. This is a conundrum, and more than being just perplexing, they are questions that reside in the core of our being.

On the Subject of Ethical Behavior

Nothing in the transcript of the two days of testimony offered more than an admission of culpability and a promise to do better in the future. Throughout the ages in medicine and medical research, matters of ethics, like those existing with the use of botulinum toxin, have been an issue. This started with the Hippocratic Oath, which can be summarized as *Primum non nocere*—"First do no harm." With this promise, the provider is the guarantor and the beneficiary is the patient or consumer. For a provider to violate the Hippocratic Oath takes omission, such as ignorance or misguided behavior, or it would be with malice, knowingly doing the wrong thing, usually for gain. To avoid either, it is the responsibility of the provider to act with ethical behavior that does no harm.

Gradually, rules were imposed on the provider in favor of the consumer. These have been levied to ensure promises are kept and as a means of protecting those who have less power and could be victims of abuse. These changes meant more control by the government, starting with new rules for food safety in 1906, in an act creating the forerunner of the current FDA. They started with food safety and continued with drug safety. After World War II, additional regulations concerning drug efficacy were established in 1960. As new policies were developed, there was still a measure of latitude in the development and marketing of drugs and in the practices of physicians, especially in clinical research. "First do no harm" was often decided by the physician, especially in areas of research, and not necessarily imposed by the authorities.

When Dr. Schantz received a request for a small amount of botulinum toxin type A or saxitoxin, he supplied researchers he knew and trusted. They used the toxin for basic research aimed at bettering the health of humankind. Though the government "owned" the toxins and there was reason to believe the authorities would approve his actions, there were no specific guidelines. Even when Dr. Schantz worked at the University of Wisconsin, he continued to act according to his own best judgment.

10

Edward Schantz Testifies

A home for botulinum toxin is determined.

A revealing government document sheds light on the question about the fate of the toxins developed at Fort Detrick. In the document, the closely guarded operation is described, and the toxin's custodian is identified. But the obligations and limits on the custodian are not established, except as described vaguely by Dr. Schantz himself and tacitly agreed to by the government. The transcript implies the whereabouts of the various toxins but falls short of establishing the provenance of botulinum toxin type A. It is mentioned only in passing during the day-long testimony provided by Dr. Schantz.

His questioners sought information that added to what they had learned on the first two days of the hearing about how the toxins had been used.[1] The senators wanted to know if the CIA disposed of poisons, and if not, how they were used, especially after the president's order had been issued. It was apparent from the questioning on the third day that the senators, guided by the chairman, aimed to do the right thing. This could have included establishing a policy that would allow useful toxins to be spared. The committee also decided to anoint a qualified custodian they trusted, Dr. Edward Schantz, to supervise the toxins. He was treated with respect, almost gently, by the senators as he testified the full day on Thursday, September 18, 1975. That day, the fate of botulinum toxin type A was decided, though mention of the toxin was only peripheral.

THE SENATE SELECT COMMITTEE HEARING

The Select Committee to Study Government Operations with Respect to Intelligence Activities was chaired by Senator Frank Church, who

characterized the session as "Puzzlement of the Poisons"—or more specifically, a discussion of the fate of toxins developed at Fort Detrick under the
aegis of the Office of Strategic Services (OSS) and CIA.[2]

The committee's sole witness this day had retired from his post at Fort
Detrick in 1971. At the time of the hearing, he was a professor at the University of Wisconsin-Madison and recognized as an expert in the field of
toxins.

The committee treated Dr. Schantz as a cooperating witness. The information he provided supported the committee's recommendation that
toxins that were useful for creating drugs to fight disease should not be destroyed. The toxin discussed in most detail was saxitoxin (shellfish toxin),
but it was not the only one spared. Others not described in detail were
implied, and this included botulinum toxin.

The transcripts of the hearing reveal that Dr. Schantz readily answered
the questions; and his replies were brief, specific, and carefully worded.
His testimony provided answers to the senators' questions without going
into more detail than necessary. He did not go out of his way to "educate"
his questioners, who were dealing with a subject mostly foreign to them.
Most of the testimony dealt with various aspects of shellfish toxin that Dr.
Schantz was willing to elaborate on. Botulinum toxin type A—including its
use, the amount produced, amount remaining, and how and when it was
shared—was never discussed.

Here is an example of Dr. Schantz saying only what he had to and nothing more. Question: "While you were there, Doctor, were you aware that
the CIA had a relationship with Fort Detrick?"[3] Answer: "Well, I did not
know that directly, now there would be a good reason to guess that, but I
did not know it at the time."

At another time, he was precise. Question: "What proportion of the
amount of shellfish toxin ever produced at any laboratory in the world is
eleven grams?"[4] Answer: "About one-third."

This was confirmed in later testimony. It meant that two-thirds of it
had been dispensed and presumably used for something, but Dr. Shantz
stated he had no records of how much was sent out or who received it.
By this time, he had given it to scientists at several facilities to test for the
presence of shellfish toxin and to make sure that safety precautions were
adhered to before selling the food. This answer was accepted. He was asked
again about shellfish toxin later, and he appeared eager to share with the
senators.

Questioned further about the lethality of shellfish toxin, Dr. Schantz replied, "It is considered an extremely lethal substance." When pressed on how much it would take to kill a human, he replied: "Two-tenths of a milligram would be sufficient." Later, a questioner asked about the shellfish toxin that remained in the Fort Detrick lab when Dr. Schantz left, and it was revealed that it would be sufficient to kill about fifty-five thousand people.[5] There was no discussion about the fate of this toxin.

A senator spoke of botulism "pills" in a jesting reference to Ian Fleming's fictional character James Bond, and botulism was mentioned one other time without comment. Later in his testimony, Dr. Schantz's only reference to the botulinum toxin was to name it in a list of other toxins. Question: "What else did you work with?" Answer: "*Clostridium botulinum* toxins, staphylococcal enterotoxins mainly, and of course shellfish poison."[6]

In his testimony, Dr. Schantz volunteered that the shellfish toxin was doled out carefully in small amounts to various laboratories in the United States, to allies like Great Britain and Canada, and to other friendly nations, "but not behind the Iron Curtain."

He said the shellfish toxins were used to prepare assays to determine their presence (or absence) in shellfish. If toxins were detected, the shellfish would not be sold but destroyed, meaning sickness and even death would be avoided. When asked specifically how much of the toxin went to the special operations division located at Fort Detrick, Dr. Schantz said he could not answer accurately but would assume that over the years they had been given "probably 10 or 15 grams."[7]

On further questioning, Dr. Schantz told the committee he provided toxins to researchers he knew worked in accredited laboratories. They were given small amounts that were specific to their research goals. When asked directly, he repeated that he did not have records of these dispersals. On further questioning, he told the committee he gave the toxin to people he knew personally or by reputation, and he would follow their work by reading reports that they published in the scientific literature.

These answers seemed to satisfy the senators. Dr. Schantz made it clear he was operating on an honor system. He dispensed the toxins as he saw fit and was not bound to comply with established rules. There were none! This kind of behavior was typical of an era in medicine when a person was given more latitude. They would be relying on their own good judgment, acting in a way they believed to be appropriate.

When the subject of the destruction of toxins came up, Dr. Schantz answered as follows: "The procedures for destruction were clear enough for me. There is no question about that. Later they were clarified and did not apply to materials for research or for public health and so forth."[8] (By 1975, he had provided Dr. Alan Scott and at least two other researchers, Dr. Vernon Brooks and Dr. Daniel Drachman, with botulinum toxin type A for basic research that impacted Scott's work. According to Dr. Eric Johnson, many others had also received the toxin.)

Senator Church then asked Dr. Schantz, "Doctor, did you serve as a custodian of the physical sciences division of the stockpile of toxin?"

Schantz answered, "Yes, I did."[9]

This was the key answer in his testimony. It confirmed Dr. Schantz was responsible for the fate of *all* toxins that were produced and dispersed, as well as those that remained when the activities of the OSS and CIA no longer called for them. It was Dr. Edward Schantz who watched over this supply of toxins, making sure it was kept safe, that it was sent out to reliable people, *and* that the toxins useful for public health and research were not destroyed. The lack of any follow-up by the senators served as tacit approval that the final authority in the matter of toxins lay with Dr. Edward Schantz.

Botulinum Toxin Type A Moves to Wisconsin

When he left Fort Detrick and headed to the University of Wisconsin, what else could Dr. Schantz do but make what he believed was the right decision regarding the fate of the toxin in his custody? There was no better solution than for the "recipe" for its production to remain with Dr. Schantz, so it went with him.

This was how he was able to provide Dr. Scott with the material after 1971 and until 1991 when the drug, then called Oculinum, was sold to Allergan. Although the direct question was not asked, the only toxin Dr. Schantz was likely to have taken with him was botulinum toxin type A. The others were left at Fort Detrick, including some of the botulinum toxin type A.

Edward Schantz did not say he destroyed the toxin when he left Fort Detrick, nor did he say how much remained or what happened to it. However, he had the recipe that allowed him to continue to produce botulinum toxin type A and he intended to continue supplying Dr. Scott. Schantz operated in a way he considered open and responsible, and the results have proved him right. The most telling part of Dr. Schantz's testimony may be when he said he did not *possess* records of how much toxin was distributed or who it went to, something that was uncharacteristic for a scientist dealing with these substances.

This statement did not mean that no records were kept. The records could be somewhere, or they could have been destroyed by someone else, and there would have been many opportunities for that. Despite this irregularity, the panel asked no further searching questions or gave any indication they needed to hear more. They were satisfied with Ed Schantz's answers and were willing to accept his judgment.

A Letter to the CIA Director

Another example of taking initiative in the story of botulinum toxin is a letter written by Committee Chair Frank Church to CIA Director William E. Colby. This letter was presented to the committee members for their signature. It had to have been written before Dr. Schantz's testimony, although its content and conclusions seemed to have been guided by what Dr. Schantz had said. Did Dr. Schantz and Senator Church meet ahead of time to discuss this testimony? Did the chairman dictate the letter during the lunch break? The letter makes it clear the chairman had already made up his own mind before the committee had the opportunity to hear in full what Dr. Schantz had to say or to discuss among themselves.

> Dear Mr. Colby:
>
> Last January, when the Select Committee was created, Senator Mansfield and Senator Scott asked that the Central Intelligence Agency not destroy any material that would relate to the committee's investigation. Biological toxins that are the subject of the committee's first public hearing are subject to the ban on destruction. The purpose of this letter is to inform you that at the completion of the committee's investigation into the improper retention by the CIA of these deadly toxins, the committee votes to approve the destruction of the toxic material in your possession.
>
> However, before the CIA proceeds to destroy these toxins we would direct your attention to the attached testimony. If adequate safety and security cautions could be taken, the committee believes that it might be appropriate for the CIA to consider donating these toxins in this [sic], consistent with our treaty obligations to properly supervised research facilities which can use these poisons for benign uses such as curing the debilitating disease such as multiple sclerosis. It is fitting that out of an admitted wrongdoing some benefit might be had. It is hoped that in this instance the committee and the executive branch can rectify past abuses and reach a mutual solution for the disposal of these lethal poisons that will be directed toward bettering the lives of our citizens.[10]

This letter indicates the committee approved Dr. Schantz's actions. If any toxin remained at Fort Detrick, it would be the responsibility of the current director. Any botulinum toxin type A retained by Dr. Schantz, including new toxin he produced, would be his responsibility. And according to the practice he had established, it would include Dr. Scott's use in his research activities in San Francisco.

At the conclusion of his testimony, nothing was said about Dr. Schantz continuing his role as custodian of the toxin nor was there any discussion about the destruction of toxin and poisons at Fort Detrick.

In the botulinum toxin type A story, Dr. Edward Schantz is a good soldier. He behaved in a responsible manner when he saved the toxin, and he continued to behave that way when he dispensed it selectively to researchers whom he believed would use it to further science. Finally, he continued to certify the high-quality toxin used for Dr. Scott's work as he completed the years of clinical trials and found a company that would take on a project originally serving the small market that included patients mostly with strabismus and dystonia (muscle spasm) around the head and neck. Edward Schantz was the right person at the right time, and he did the right thing.

11

Back in Madison

Without fanfare, Edward Schantz continued his role as custodian of the culture of botulinum toxin type A, but now he had the approval of the United States Senate.

The course for both Schantz and the toxin was settled.

Edward Schantz's professional career was a paradox. He began as a farmer and food researcher. In a second phase, he worked with deadly toxins for nearly three decades in the Army Chemical Research Facility as an officer and later as a civilian employee. Finally, he returned to food research, where he also carried out an important supporting role in the development of a drug for humans. It would come from the deadly toxin he had spent a major part of his career taming. It would now find a better use.[1]

A characteristic of this man was his even-handed behavior and genuine kindness that, according to Dr. Eric Johnson, a long-time collaborator, was an unfailing feature of his senior colleague.[2] Another young researcher, Dr. Daniel Drachman, met Ed Schantz for the first time in 1962 and marveled at the kind and gentle demeanor of this man who dealt with "the deadliest of all toxins."[3]

Ed Schantz remained at the University of Wisconsin until his second retirement twenty years later. By 1984, Schantz was working regularly with Dr. Johnson. The two produced, tested, and conducted assays on the botulinum toxin type A culture while ensuring that the toxin they dispensed was of the highest quality.

Dr. Johnson recalled: "The pattern was like this: I would be working in my office with my own projects in the morning and Doctor Schantz would come by. He would ask me if I had some time this morning and I always said yes. We would spend about four hours in his lab doing various things and talking about anything that interested us. He was a kind man. He was nice to everybody, and I rarely saw him angry."[4]

The essence of Schantz's far-reaching contribution can be recognized in no better way than through his willingness and encouragement in helping others. One of the first researchers he assisted was also a person whose life was impacted by the events of World War II, which was at the center of much of what has been depicted here. Werner Bruck was born in Berlin, Germany, in 1923. Ten years later, when Adolf Hitler became chancellor, the young man's tranquil life was changed. In his words, "Although we had no religious life, we were considered Jews by the government. Generations of cultural assimilation, fervor, patriotism, and service as an officer in World War I had come to mean nothing in my father's case."

In 1938, his family sent young Werner to Britain for his own safety. There, according to prior arrangement, he was put in the care of a local family in Kent, England. He completed his primary education and emigrated to Canada. Noting that the locals pronounced his name Bruck as "truck" and that it was painful to his ears, he took the new surname Brooks and changed Werner to Vernon. He earned his PhD in physiology in 1952 and specialized in neurophysiology. According to Dr. Brooks, "Later I discovered that I had been an inadvertent godfather for the Botox treatment of many dystonias and other involuntary muscle movements."

How did this happen?

This statement by Brooks was explained in a symposium book, *Therapy with Botulinum Toxin*, in a footnote quotation by Edward Schantz. Schantz explained, "The possible use of Botulinum toxin for weakening a muscle was first suggested to me by Doctor Vernon Brooks a physiologist I had provided with toxin in the early 50s for his studies. Dr. Brooks [supported by the work of A. S. Burgen and Arthur Guyton] said he had shown that the toxin blocked acetylcholine released to the muscles, and he suggested in the 1950s that the toxin would be good to reduce the activity of hyperactive muscles."[5]

According to Dr. Johnson, with the botulinum toxin back at Wisconsin, some went to supply Dr. Daniel Drachman, whose important work had begun in the 1960s. When a productive researcher was asking for more, Ed Schantz continued to offer support. After 1972, this included Alan Scott and led to an extended relationship. During this time an agreement was reached with the university whose policy did not include supporting research carried out expressly for commercial purposes. In Alan Scott's case it was decided his primary goal was to find answers to scientific questions.

The commercial success with botulinum toxin came later, not by design, and provided little more than a return of capital for the developers.

Alan Scott learned about Dr. Drachman's work and Dr. Schantz in a round-about way. Dr. Edward Maumenee, then chairman of the Wilmer Institute of Ophthalmology at Johns Hopkins Hospital, knew about Drachman be-cause he was a neurologist at the hospital, and he was also familiar with botulinum toxin because Maumenee was briefly associated with a project dealing with the toxin when he was a naval officer during World War II, stationed for a short time at Camp Detrick.[6]

Dr. Maumenee's first assignment as a new officer in the navy was to join a group studying the possibility of the Germans poisoning England's water supply with botulinum toxin. According to Maumenee, the team de-cided that this would be impractical, and it was highly unlikely this type of warfare would ever be conducted. He also said he was not interested in this assignment and was pleased when he moved on to new duty on a hos-pital ship in the Pacific. Maumenee's most memorable recollection about his involvement with the toxin at Camp Detrick was that he injected it into a chicken's eye and the pupil dilated. This could be useful to determine the presence of the toxin, but it was not an easy test to perform.

Around 1972, Ed Maumenee, who had been director of the ophthal-mology section at Stanford and a colleague of Arthur Jampolsky, told him about Daniel Drachman, who, like Scott, was a rising young researcher. The difference in the launch of these careers could hardly be greater. Drach-man had done all his work in prestigious eastern institutions with highly regarded mentors. Scott was working in a small laboratory, just getting started and benefiting from helpful advice from his mentor in residency training and from two basic scientists skilled in neuroscience. They were willing to help a young colleague just starting his career as a researcher. In contrast, Dr. Drachman was using botulinum toxin in the laboratory that he was developing in a prestigious institution. Jampolsky passed on this information to Scott, who contacted Drachman, who unselfishly shared knowledge in an example of "handed down" information, as was common in the research community.[7]

Dr. Daniel Drachman, in the book celebrating the fiftieth anniversary of the Neuromuscular Division of the Department of Neurology at Johns Hopkins that bears his name, said, "That's how Botox really got discovered:

68   Death to Beauty

Alan Scott, an ophthalmologist in San Francisco wanted to use it for strabismus so he called me and asked me how to do it."[8] (Claiming discovery can be a slippery slope. Vernon Brooks had injected botulinum toxin into a muscle nearly ten years earlier, and it produced weakness, which led to him being called by some the "godfather of Botox.")

Drachman's claim is supported by his report on the result of injecting botulinum toxin into one leg of a chicken embryo, causing underdevelopment of muscles from lack of innervation during development. This experiment was an important step in learning more about the causes of the commonly occurring congenital condition called clubfoot. Drachman's groundbreaking work in explaining the events leading to this condition was key, but the effects of the toxin injected into a mature muscle in a human would not be described for another decade.[9]

A Common Path for Researchers

The work ethic and ingenuity displayed by Dr. Daniel Drachman at the outset of his research career is remarkably like two other medical doctors / teachers / researchers who also played a prominent role in the botulinum toxin story: Arthur Guyton at Camp Detrick and Alan Scott at the Smith-Kettlewell Eye Research Institute. Each began working in a new lab that lacked suitable equipment to begin their scientific projects. Each needed a way to record the electrical activity associated with nerve transmission to muscles. And all three met the challenge in a similar way: they designed, assembled, and learned to operate equipment based on their own ingenuity. In each case, it worked. All made significant contributions toward understanding botulinum toxin that contributed to its eventual use in a human. These men were physicians with different specialties. They were a physiologist, a neurologist, and an ophthalmologist / strabismologist. In this way they were unique, but all shared the skill and tenacity that led to success.

As a scientist working to learn more about disease process, Drachman was not impressed with Scott's plans that could have been interpreted as having a commercial aim. Later Drachman lamented, partly in jest, "I should have patented that and I would be billions of dollars ahead."[10]

For his part, Scott was not in search of a patent for his work with botulinum toxin, at least initially, but the Smith-Kettlewell Institute would have welcomed it as would Scott later when he tried to sell Oculinum to a pharmaceutical company. Early in the course of his work, Scott, who published carefully and with consequence, had explained the action of botulinum toxin. This was in a paper published in 1973 that described the first use of the toxin in a primate. This disclosure ruled out any possibility of obtaining a patent![12] (Publicly disclosing an idea before submitting its patent application is one of the most common ways of compromising the patentability of an invention. In fact, once an idea is publicly disclosed, such ideas become prior art of the invention, and therefore the invention will no longer meet the novelty requirement.)

After speaking with Drachman about botulinum toxin and determining how his research efforts could benefit from these useful pointers, Scott contacted Ed Schantz in April 1972. He did this in a letter where he inquired about receiving the toxin for his work on weakening extraocular muscles to develop a targeted nonsurgical technique to treat strabismus.

THE THREAD OF KNOWLEDGE

Schantz supplied Scott with the toxin and also passed on important information he had learned from other researchers he had helped. He told Scott about Brooks' earlier discovery and about the work of Arnold Burgen and Arthur Guyton. At Camp Detrick, Guyton had been the first to advance a theory explaining the role of acetylcholine at the neuromuscular junction. And he provided electromyographic evidence that demonstrated how botulinum toxin could affect muscle action. This provided evidence that demonstrated botulinum toxin could be useful for targeted weakening of overactive muscles in a primate, with an effect that lasted months. This important information only reinforced what Scott had learned from Drachman. Scott was encouraged.

Alan Scott's work that was supported by the information passed along to him by Ed Schantz and others is an example of how scientific discoveries build in importance over time. Each contributor in the botulinum toxin story benefits from the prior work of others, adds new information, and freely passes on the fruits of their own labor. People who can share only through what they leave behind for others to pick up and use have been with us through history. They are like the cathedral builders who toiled for generations building an edifice stone by stone and leaving their own work for future generations to complete it and view the finished product.

This is a recurring theme in the story of botulinum toxin, as researchers shared what they learned—unselfishly and with pride.

Here is the text of the letter recording Alan Scott's first contact with Dr. Schantz. It was generously shared by Dr. Eric Johnson:

April 17, 1972

Dear Doctor Schantz,

Through the publications of Doctor Drachman, I understand botulinum toxin may be available from you for experimental use. It is our intent to paralyze individual extraocular muscles by injection directly into the muscle in the region of the myoneural junction in order to [*sic*] study the function of the ocular motor system after ablation of functions without inferring with the anatomic tissues themselves by surgical techniques.

I shall be grateful for your help and suggestions as to apply safety matters and utilization of the material. Thank you very much.

Sincerely,
Alan B. Scott

12

Dr. Alan B. Scott

A regular kid who grew up in Northern California.

"Not everyone who moved to California during the Gold Rush planned to earn a fortune by using a pan or a pickaxe in the goldfields. Many enterprising young men and women realized there was just as much money to be made by providing the goldminers with goods and services. From professional men and merchants to dancehall girls and card sharks, they gave the miners a way to spend their money. In addition, many who came to mine gold found that business and farming in California were a more satisfying and reliable source of income."[1]

This was a fair description of three young men who set out for California from the East Coast in 1849 to seek their fortune. These men were the forebears of Dr. Alan B. Scott. The travelers were forward-looking and resourceful men who had saved nearly a year of wages each to make the eight-month, fifteen-thousand-mile trip around Cape Horn to this new state and new life. The men had a stake and a plan that could have included mining but there is no evidence this was their principal aim.

On the outward leg, one of the brothers decided to get off at Panama. He was a bright fellow who had been a translator for the government, and he did some business on the isthmus then made his way overland to meet his two brothers after they had gone around the tip of South America. They reconnected flawlessly on the Pacific side, and the three men continued to their destination.

Once in San Francisco, two of the brothers decided to visit an establishment that offered refreshments and entertainment. The third brother was stationed outside with the responsibility of watching their stash. There is no record of what that stash contained, but the contents must have been important. When the two brothers rejoined the third to retrieve what they had left, they were told it was gone, and the brother who had been assigned to guard it had no ready explanation.

Alan Scott recounted this family lore. He added that the two disappointed young men never spoke to their brother again. Instead, they turned to farming to become the foundation of the Scott family. He finished the comment with a chuckle, saying, "I don't know if that is true, but that's what I have been told."[2]

This story of the young men who planted the Scott family in California set a high bar for persistence and pluck, which turned out to have a lasting effect that would shine clearly in the twenty-first-century man who was sharing his family history.

* * *

Three generations later, in San Francisco, a young woman, working as a lab technician, was urged to continue her education in the field of science. The man trying to convince her was Dr. Karl Meyer, a Swiss research scientist who was both a veterinarian and immunologist.[3] He held positions at both the University of California Berkeley and the University of California San Francisco, where he established a department of bacteriology and later joined the Hooper Foundation, which he headed for twenty-one years.

Meyer's first job at the foundation was to build a team to study botulinum toxin and find a way to eliminate the scourge of botulism poisoning that threatened the burgeoning local canning industry in 1919. The producers were trying to restore confidence in their canned food after olives contaminated with botulinum toxin caused more than two dozen deaths nationwide. Meyer, who continued a brilliant career spanning forty years, eventually succeeded in both efforts.

Leading a group of scientists, Karl Meyer devised guidelines and established manufacturing practices to destroy *Clostridium botulinum* spores during the canning process. His work bolstered confidence that helped save California's commercial canning industry. Supported by these efforts, canned foods from the state could now be marketed with confidence that they were safe for consumption.

This scientist had also been successful in convincing the young woman to become a microbiologist, but there is no evidence she joined his team. As it turned out, the young woman, Helen Elizabeth Scott (née Brown), would also have a part in the botulinum toxin story. However, it would be through her son, Alan Brown Scott, who one day carried out his unique role in that story—not only in the state but also in the world.

Helen had no way to suspect her son would someday be a pioneer in his own way. Alan Brown Scott would be the first person to inject the world's deadliest toxin in a human in 1978 for the purpose of treating misalignment of the eyes. After that, he would achieve stunning success—while working on his own—developing a new drug that would eventually treat millions worldwide and launch a multibillion-dollar industry for Botox.

YOUNG ALAN SCOTT

Alan Brown Scott was born in Berkeley, California, on July 13, 1932. He had an older sister, and they were close. According to Scott, his parents were supportive but not demanding. His mother continued to work in microbiology, and his father was a dentist. "My parents were good people," Scott told me during one of several conversations he and I had in 2021.

He attended Cragmont Elementary School, Berkeley High School, and the University of California at Berkeley. All of these were in his hometown, Berkeley, a community of eighty thousand, located north of Oakland and east of San Francisco across the bay. In high school, he played clarinet in the band. The rest of the time he went to school and, in his own words with a smile, "chased the girls and just had fun." He spent summers on a local fruit farm, usually working ten hours a day. Because he was tall for his age, young Alan had no trouble getting a driver's license before he was fourteen. With a license, he was able to drive the truck on the farm, and that made him a more valuable contributor.

Two things about this man that stood out when we talked were Scott's enthusiasm and his love for work. In the beginning, this mostly centered around working summers in the orchard. "Oh, and I almost forgot to mention during the summer I had time off from college. My sister and her husband, who was in the army stationed in Alaska, invited me to stay with them when school was out. I spent two summers there, working construction as a union iron worker."

There was something about school he did not disclose but I learned later. Scott earned Phi Beta Kappa after three years. This is a high honor to earn as a junior. He left his undergraduate life at the University of California, Berkeley early when he was accepted into medical school. He did not mention this award. How Alan Scott viewed himself, I was learning, depended on accomplishments he could claim as his own, not on honors bestowed by others.

His comments on the University of California, Berkeley, which he was obviously proud of attending, included, "Some say it is number one, but others say it's number thirty. Take your choice." When asked about his major, he said after a pause, "I guess it was premed, but I didn't finish, because I was accepted into medical school early." He added, "I lived at home about half-time and in a fraternity the rest. The tuition was forty-nine dollars a semester."

"When did you decide on medicine?" I asked him.

"I don't know. I could have been a farmer, but becoming a doctor just fell together."

Alan Scott said this while giving the clear impression that work for him was not just a job, it was a way of life that he sought.

Alan and Ruth Scott were married in 1956, the year of his graduation from medical school at the University of San Francisco. They eventually had five children. A daughter is a physician practicing obstetrics and gynecology in Oregon. Scott said, "The others do all sorts of things, some pretty interesting. They are all nice kids." He was continuing to express himself as a master of understatement.

After graduating from medical school, Scott's career path took him to Minnesota, far from his familiar haunts in Berkeley. This move turned out to be the only venture that found him temporarily veering off course, geographically if not medically. What lured this California native to one of the coldest cities in the country? The answer was it happened to be the location of one of the two best cardiac surgery programs in the United States. (The other was in Houston.) Alan Scott's aim was to become a heart surgeon!

The Minnesota program was led by renowned surgeon Dr. Owen Wangensteen, and a leader in the new field of open-heart surgery, C. Walton Lillehei, directed a team working in the operating room and the laboratory. With these two luminaries, Minnesota was clearly first in Scott's mind. An example of the type of person recruited by the program was Dr. Christiaan Barnard, a rising star in the field who later developed the world's first artificial heart in Cape Town, South Africa. His presence only added luster to this star-studded department.

But a growing family, the prospect of spending four years in the laboratory before beginning clinical work, and an insistent Ruth made Alan decide to switch. Neurosurgery was the next choice for his training path, as it meant he would continue at the same university in a different department. For largely the same reasons, this did not work either. His next decision stuck. He headed back to California to train in ophthalmology at Stanford.

Once back home, Alan Scott, comfortable as a fourth-generation Californian, resumed life in familiar surroundings. He completed ophthalmology training at Stanford and remained in the San Francisco area. Everything fell into place for Alan and Ruth. It turned out this decision was a good one. After this, the only times he would leave the Bay Area were for vacation or to travel to a medical meeting. Scott knew where he wanted to be. This decision also meant he would never be far from his original medical office and the laboratory that gave birth to the successful drug he would eventually develop.

Though Stanford ophthalmology was not at the relative level of prominence as the heart team in Minnesota, there was a solid core of teachers in the program. The retina surgeon Dorman Pischell headed it. "I could have decided on being a retina surgeon, but Dr. Pischell refused to use the new indirect ophthalmoscope, so I dropped that idea," said Scott. (This was a new binocular head-mounted device that enabled a more complete examination of the back of the eye. Since it took a period of adjustment to get used to it, many established practitioners eschewed this device in favor of the less effective but familiar handheld monocular scope. The indirect scope soon became the standard.)

When the Stanford ophthalmology residency training program shifted the third year of training from Palo Alto to San Francisco, Dr. Scott was allowed more freedom. After his clinic duties were completed, he spent three months each with three of his old Stanford teachers who practiced in San Francisco.

Dr. Arthur Jampolsky, one of the three faculty under whom Scott studied, was thirteen years senior and had been in practice in San Francisco for six years. Prior to medical school, this outgoing, gap-toothed, and seldom in doubt on any subject ophthalmologist had trained as an optometrist. Smart and hardworking, Jampolsky maintained an interest in optics and the study of the action of the extraocular muscles. He was developing a new research laboratory to study visual science, and that interested Alan Scott.

Earlier, Dr. Jampolsky had spent two months in Sweden visiting the Karolinska Institute, a research-led medical school in Stockholm that is rated near the best in the world. There he was exposed to basic science techniques. His time spent abroad at a world-famous institution added panache to Jampolsky's ideas for research and to his lab, the Smith-Kettlewell Eye Research Institute. Visiting prestigious institutions and colleagues in Europe to broaden medical and scientific experience was a common practice for physicians from the United States, beginning in the nineteenth century. Alan Scott had found a mentor with a lab and a purpose. This was an attractive opportunity, but there were alternatives. It was time for Scott to decide where to start practice. Key in the process was how he would shape that activity so he could function as a healer and still satisfy his need to find answers to the many unanswered questions already encountered in his time in training. Scott had an active mind and wanted to stretch it.

With a growing family and his ophthalmology training nearing the end, important decisions loomed for Alan and Ruth. Key among these was where to set up his practice. Scott knew there was an opportunity for an ophthalmologist to go just about anywhere in the state and, in his words, "earn a handsome living." But he said, "I realized this could be pretty boring; that's why I decided to stay in town." This decision was characteristic of Alan Scott's attitude throughout life. He put almost everything ahead of simply making more money. Instead, he made decisions based on making the most of the life he chose to live.

Scott's decision could be said to have created a paradox. He was able to accomplish something even bigger when he resisted the lure of pulling up stakes and spreading his wings to forge a new path. By staying home, in familiar surroundings that were comfortable and productive, he remained in contact with colleagues and mentors, and he maintained professional ties that were accessible and trusted. Scott marshaled his energy and enthusiasm to accomplish his special interests as he built on an already established foundation. It was not necessary to start from scratch, but there was much still to be done, and this is something he relished.

As an added incentive for the Scott family, what better place was there to live in the 1960s than the San Francisco area? He decided to pursue a career in the place where he was born, educated, and started his family. In doing so, Alan Scott led a professional life that had a global impact unsurpassed by any of his peers. He spent his working life, for the most part, within fifty miles of where he was born. In this mode, his life would not be consumed by dealing with *where* he was but instead *who* he was and *what* he accomplished. These familiar surroundings supplied all he needed to proceed with his plans and allowed him freedom to work in a place where he was both productive and comfortable. There was no grand plan laying this all out, but as Scott's life and career unfolded, it turned out he did not have to take his show "on the road." He stayed home and gained worldwide fame.

In the beginning, Scott was influenced by a range of clinical research schemes shared by his mentor, Art Jampolsky. These ideas were broad in scope but needed focus before getting started. This array offered an inviting challenge. In 1961, starting with little more than a nudge, Scott began work in the lab and plotted a course he would pursue relentlessly. With help and encouragement from two basic scientists, Carter Collins III and David Robinson, on an informal basis, and a laboratory for his use, Scott was poised for action.

When asked how he had narrowed the options, he said, "We hit on . . . exploring the forces and actions of eye muscles." This morphed into "injecting local anesthetic into individual muscles to knock out their function and to tell thereby what they did. It was a small step to wonder if we could inject something having a longer duration of action and thus practical utility." He was searching for a newer and better way to treat crossed eyes.

First, Scott needed to learn all he could about how the eye muscles worked. Then his task was to find the answer to these key questions: How can an eye muscle's action be controlled as it affects an opposing muscle in the same eye and others in the fellow eye as they guide images from the optic nerve to the brain? Does the sensory part of the brain that registers a single image exert control on eye muscles and alignment in selected cases of misalignment called *strabismus*?

Scott's goal was to find a way to treat misalignment of the eyes by temporarily weakening the action of an extraocular muscle in one or both eyes, thereby altering the way the muscles reacted with each other. This would balance the muscle forces on the eyes with the aim of straightening them. This could improve appearance and possibly function. In some cases, it was hoped the brain could guide the eyes toward perfect alignment and single binocular vision, or close to it. Earlier attempts at doing this by others, as well as Scott, with a variety of agents, were unsuccessful.[4] The time was right for a novel approach.

Before Scott could begin his research to realign the eyes without resorting to traditional incisional surgery, there was work to do. He realized that before fixing something, one must know precisely what is not working properly. There was preliminary work to be done. In the summer of 1961, Scott began work each morning in the lab plotting a course he pursued relentlessly throughout his long career in medicine. In the afternoon he saw patients and performed surgery in the operating room.

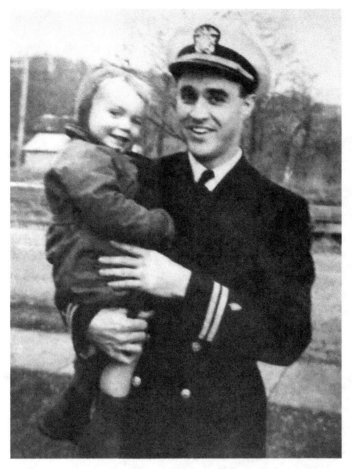

Arthur Guyton, age 27, holding son David in 1946, the first of ten Guyton children, all of whom became medical doctors. (Used by permission.)

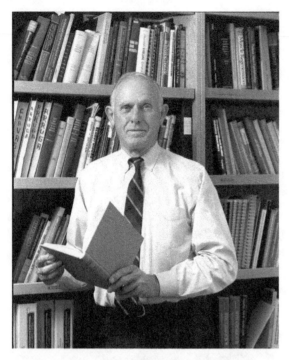

Alan Brown Scott, developer of Botox (July 13, 1932–December 16, 2021). (Courtesy of the Smith-Kettlewell Eye Research Institute.)

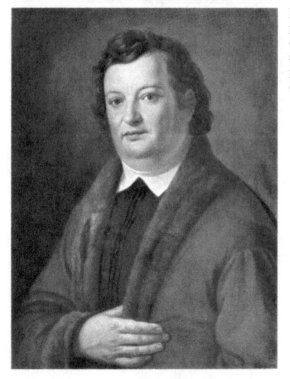

Justinus Kerner (1786–1862) predicted in 1822 that the death-dealing toxin from blood sausage could have a medicinal purpose. (Courtesy of Wikimedia Commons.)

An example of Kerner klecksography, with subtle additions making it appear something like a butterfly. (Courtesy of Wikimedia Commons.)

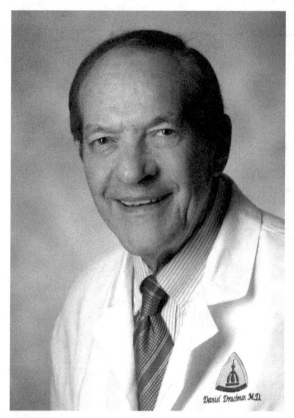

Left: Daniel Drachman from Johns Hopkins provided early support to Alan Scott in dealing with botulinum toxin. (Used by permission.)

Below: Dr. Edward Schantz in his lab at the Wisconsin Food Safety Institute with Dr. Eric Johnson looking on. (Courtesy of the University of Wisconsin Archives.)

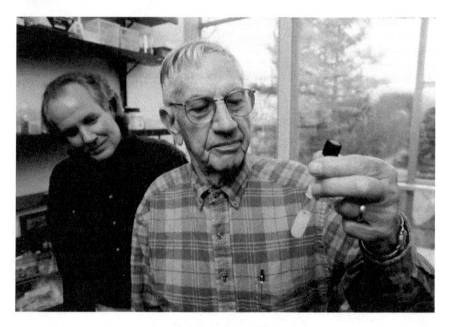

13

Progress in the Lab

Scott's work in the laboratory began immediately.

Starting his ophthalmology practice, Scott spent time daily in the laboratory his mentor had established. In the lab he worked beside mostly full-time researchers who pursued their own interests independently while delving into the visual sciences, an interest Scott shared. As a clinician practicing in a private office, each afternoon Scott found himself with a foot solidly planted across the divide separating basic science and clinical practice. He started in an independent lab established by his mentor Art Jampolsky that by 1963 became the San Francisco Eye Research Institute. In 1969 it was renamed the Smith-Kettlewell Eye Research Institute, an independent research facility named for two benefactors Jampolsky had engaged in this effort. The lab later established academic standing by associating with the California Pacific Medical Center. Scott was comfortable splitting his time between the lab and seeing patients in his private office, sacrificing income for the enticement of research.

"My first year in practice, I made twelve thousand dollars. That was more in those days compared to now, but it still wasn't much, and we had to be imaginative," he said with a smile.[1]

The atmosphere and the people associated with the lab, according to Scott, exuded enthusiasm and esprit. In the beginning, it was a congenial atmosphere that was both supportive and open to new ideas—a great place to start for a person on a mission.

One of the financial backers of the new lab was Clement J. Smith. He was described by Scott as a brilliant daredevil enthralled with visions of astounding feats, who often showed off by saying things like "I'm a bird!" and then pretending to fly.

Adding to the hometown touch, Scott said his father had raced against Smith in high school track meets, and that Smith was a character even then. Smith became wealthy after a stint in China, where he connected with Cornelius Vander Starr, who turned American Asiatic Underwriters into one of the most successful insurance companies in the world. He later named the company American International Group (AIG). William A. Kettlewell, the other benefactor, was a successful dam builder in California and later in postwar Japan. Scott, who was usually more grounded in his answers, seemed to take pleasure in describing the character of these offbeat benefactors whose actions might have lent an avant-garde luster to the institute that bore their name.

Both Smith and Kettlewell had family members with eye health problems. Arthur Jampolsky provided ongoing help to both; in gratitude, each provided initial funding and continued support for the institute that still functions with their mission: "To create a unique environment for research on human vision."[2]

Starting at Smith-Kettlewell, Alan Scott was eager to take up a project that was already in the beginning stages but existed mostly in the form of ideas with challenges. Arthur Jampolsky, based on interests developed in his prior training in eyecare, encouraged his young associate to use electromyography to learn more about the mechanics and physiology of eye movement. This fits perfectly with Alan Scott's wish to explore the mysteries of eye muscle action, eye movement, and overall neural control, but it would take more than wishing, it took doing. This planning was important, but things did not "just happen." There were techniques to learn and equipment to design and fabricate that were necessary to carry out the experiments that were planned. These tasks were taken on by Scott with relish.

When asked when his love of the lab began to take off, Alan's answer was, "Right away. I stayed in town, practiced in my own office, and worked closely with Art Jampolsky. Things worked out well from the start, and this is what I wanted to do."

The following, in Alan Scott's words, describes what was on his mind as he started work in the laboratory.

"In the 1960s, the outcome of strabismus surgery was far from perfect—as many as forty percent of patients needed reoperation.[3] No one knew the strength of the muscle, how much it contributed to the eye movement, what the nerve control signal provided, what parts of the muscle contracted, and so on. With a brilliant engineer, Carter Collins III, PhD, and a team to construct mechanical and electrical apparatus, we set out to make these measurements on humans and construct a rational model to guide strabismus surgery at Smith-Kettlewell, the eye research lab at California Pacific Medical Center.

"Soon I was doing a lot of things, including administration around the lab. I began as assistant director and then was made codirector. Eventually, with Art interested in things like making Fresnel membrane prisms, I was pretty much the head of the lab up through the nineties. After that, we had a readjustment, and I spent less time at the Institute. Art and I had a falling out, but that's another story.

"In the lab, we were measuring muscle response evidenced by electrical activity from the nerve's stimulation of the muscle, electromyography (EMG). This was the kind of work begun in New York by Dr. Goodwin Briennin. He was working like us as an ophthalmologist/strabismologist. Some work like this was also being done in Europe, and interest was picking up here because need for this information was increasing on the heels of advanced techniques in diagnostics and treatment."

This work by Scott and his team was state-of-the-art and served as a launching pad for later work with botulinum toxin. More than a dozen other investigators were busy in the lab, working in their own areas of interests, such as low vision, application of prism technology, binocular vision, strabismus, and more. Carter Collins was a major contributor to Alan Scott's work in the beginning. Collins was a bioengineer whom Scott described as "sort of an astronaut before astronauts." He was involved in designing gravity sleds (testing the effect of gravitational pressure on pilots) in the early days of the space program. Collins introduced David Robinson, who was also a PhD, to the team. He was studying the midbrain at Johns Hopkins, where he devised a way to program eye movements from an engineering standpoint. This had been tried earlier by an engineer from Salt Lake City, whose daughter had five surgeries, but his results were only approximate. Robinson's programs were superb, according to Scott, and they have endured as a landmark accomplishment that has been carried on by Dr. Joel Miller.

TESTING EYE MUSCLES

To move ahead with their EMG studies, Scott described how, in one of their projects, he and his group went to the California State Prison located in Vacaville, east of San Francisco. There were twenty-five hundred male inmates; many had strabismus, and most turned out to be willing subjects. "The team set up temporary labs and attached instruments to eye muscles on awake patients to measure forces and electrical activity during eye movement," Scott explained. "This wasn't that painful, but messing with your eyes was not something most people could easily withstand. Still, the prisoners were model subjects. Many of them required surgery to straighten their eyes, and surgery for them, of course, was provided free. The inmates were pleased to work with the research team and sorry to see the program end."

After a pause Dr. Scott added, "There was this big guy who could pick me up with one finger if I so much as hurt him, but he was gentle as a lamb. These fellows had been good subjects. It was a good thing for several months, and then we had to stop."

This human research project that provided a wealth of useful information, according to Alan Scott, started with optimism and concluded on a positive note.

When I asked how his lab became famous for developing Teflon-coated recording needles for EMG, Dr. Scott said, "Along the way, there was a need to find out how the muscles were contracting and so forth. The neurosurgeons and neurophysiologist were working with recordings of the brain and other nerves and were using sticky needles. They used this kind because they had to stay in place. Needles like this were not suitable for muscles, so I developed one with a tightly fitted Teflon sleeve. They are now used widely today, especially for large-muscle injections of Botox, but they are used in only ten to twenty percent of eye muscle injections." (In many instances, developing an instrument or device resulted in appending the developer's name. These could have been "Scott needles," but this was not Alan Scott's style.)

As Alan Scott talked about his journey with botulinum toxin, it was easy to imagine I was listening to him as he would speak while early in his career and just beginning this long journey. Scott must have presented as a tall, angular towhead as a young man, who spoke softly and with a twang— call it California—as he chose his words carefully. He does not strike one as a person who would change much. He was what he was. Though never appearing to be in a hurry, he seemed to be always moving forward—usually in the right direction.

"Alan Scott was the person you would choose to be in charge if you were on a hike in the woods or approaching a challenging task," said Dr. Elbert Magoon, one of Scott's students and later associate in the 1980s. "Alan is the kind of guy you just know can get the job done. You trust him."

These characteristics are not the kind to be newly acquired. They are "baked in the cake" and only perfected with time.[4]

Learning How the Muscles Work

Once the recording apparatus and techniques were established, it was time to begin learning more about how the eye muscles worked as they supported binocular vision in the human. The first task for the team was to establish a relationship and a working order between the following three entities: eye muscle, eyes, and brain. The team began with what was already known:

There are twelve extraocular muscles, six in each eye. Each muscle has an antagonist (opposite pulling) muscle in the same eye and a yoked (move together) muscle in the fellow eye.

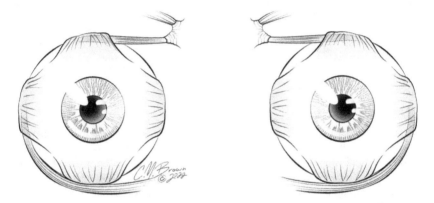

Twelve extraocular muscles move the eyes. Six are attached to each eye and present as mirror images. Each eye has a muscle to move the eye in toward the nose, up toward the eyebrow, down toward the lip, and out toward the ear. Each eye also has an upper oblique muscle that moves the eye down and rotates it in and a lower oblique muscle that pulls the eye up and rotates the eye outward.

The eyes move together and gaze in a parallel direction, except when they don't. This is shown in the bottom row of the illustration where the eyes are pointing inward to look at a near object. The aim of the yoked muscles is to have both eyes looking at the same thing. Our eyes move motorwise, as on a universal joint transmitting power over a limited range of angles. When we look at distant objects, this movement keeps the eyes working together for approximately twenty degrees in any direction in the frontal plane. For near objects that are less than twenty feet away, the eyes converge an appropriate amount to maintain the object of regard as a single image sent to the brain.

The eyes rotate precisely for distance viewing, and in a more complicated way for near, thanks to the interaction of six pairs of yoked muscles.

When looking up and down, "cooperating" muscles that are not yoked function in a way that adds more complexity to the process and must be dealt with in calculations. All these movements are on a continuum that requires precision at every point to maintain constant single binocular vision.

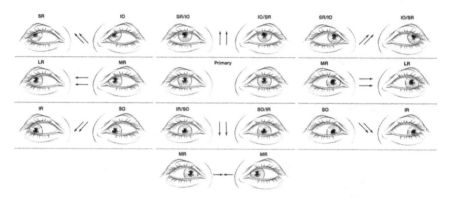

In the primary position, front-facing eyes in a human are normally "straight." When they move from this position, they work together and are parallel, viewing the same object at a distance over a range of more than 20 degrees in each direction from vision straight ahead. This results in a single image seen stereoscopically (with depth). For near vision at less than twenty feet, the eyes converge an appropriate amount to keep the object seen as one.

At its very back in an area called the *occipital cortex*, the brain registers sight from each eye and blends an overlapping image so that one object is seen in depth. In persons with aligned eyes, images just off the center of vision and more so in the periphery are seen with some disparity. This turns out to be beneficial because it enables a person using both eyes to see these images as one image with the three-dimensional perception of depth.

The aim of the Smith-Kettlewell team, led by Scott, was to determine in more detail how these muscles did their job in concert with the brain. Initially accurate recordings were completed in subjects with correctly aligned eyes. Then measurements were made in patients who had imbalanced eye muscles due to disparate contraction or mechanical restriction that caused strabismus (misaligned eyes). Measurements in patients with strabismus would define the problem to be fixed.

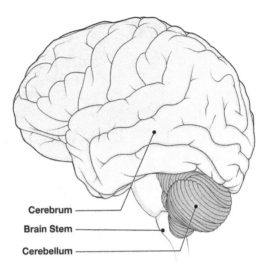

The image from each eye is registered in the back of the brain (cerebrum) in the visual cortex. There images from each eye are fused with a slight disparity producing a simultaneous perspective of a single object now seen in depth. This fusion mechanism of the brain in turn provides a signal affecting muscle function to maintain precise alignment on the object.

Cerebrum

Brain Stem

Cerebellum

Scott's goal was to find a way to treat strabismus using injection of an agent into a single or sometimes two extraocular muscles. This would be done instead of traditional incisional surgery. An earlier researcher attempted a similar injection with alcohol, but it was unsuccessful. Scott wanted to do something like this, but in a way that worked. According to Scott's plan, when the contracting power of a muscle that is doing too much and causing strabismus is reduced, the opposite (antagonist) muscle could regain strength and be more effective, at least in a relative way at first. The question was: could this change become permanent? If so, realignment of the eyes could be achieved without the need for surgery. In select cases, he hoped the brain, after receiving a more nearly aligned visual input, could lock in to achieve a single binocular image and maintain aligned eyes. This is a blend of physiology, anatomy, biochemistry, and just plain clinical know-how that would alter conditions and help the brain put things as they should be. It bridged a gap between the bench scientist in the laboratory and the clinician seeking a way to deliver a therapeutic result.

Local anesthetics were found to have too short a duration. In Scott's words, "We might inject something having a longer duration of action and thus practical utility. Botulinum toxin soon came up for consideration but was moved to the bottom of the list, as it seemed too crazy to try it. It was too toxic, and we would never get away with it with the FDA looking."

But that would change.

14

First Injection in a Primate

Botulinum toxin type A becomes the agent of choice.

With a better understanding of how the extraocular muscles worked, based on experiments and observations that spanned nearly a decade, it was time to move on. Scott's next step was to find a suitable injectable substance that would reduce the power of an eye muscle to create (or restore) proper eye alignment in a person with strabismus. (Strabismus is an abnormal appearance of the eyes and is sometimes called *squint*.) That was his focus and wished-for endpoint, which would be achieved because of the work he had already done.

Scott studied the eyes of patients with normal eye movement and alignment, as well as those with strabismus. This was supplemented by studies in cooperative subjects using minimally invasive, harmless techniques. The next step was to find and evaluate a substance that would produce targeted and long-lasting weakening of an extraocular muscle. This relied on laboratory studies, starting with mice, cats, and other small animals. Finally, to demonstrate the toxin was safe in a human, it would be necessary to conduct testing in a primate. This was the next big step.

At first, different agents injected to weaken the eye and skeletal muscles of small animals proved to be too toxic or had too short an effect. It was necessary to look further, and this led Scott to consider the possibility of using botulinum toxin. Should he take the chance? The answer came from Art Jampolsky, who had learned about the toxin being used safely in the laboratory from Dr. Edward Maumenee, chairman of the Wilmer Eye Institute at Johns Hopkins.

In 1972, the chain of discovery led Alan Scott to Daniel Drachman, a neurologist and researcher a year younger, working at Johns Hopkins. Dr.

Drachman had used botulinum toxin in his laboratory for more than a decade and shared his experience freely. It was reassuring to Scott to hear from this experienced researcher, who explained techniques for dilution, dosage, and key safety measures. Drachman later disclosed that he was not excited about the long-term prospects for this project but was more than willing to help Scott get started by offering the best advice he could.[1]

Drachman had demonstrated in his chick-embryo studies that the toxin could be like a sharp knife. He injected it into one leg and observed a profound effect in the muscle of that leg, but no other disturbance elsewhere in the embryo. He described a molecule (toxin) like a knife that cut unfailingly, doing just what was wanted and nothing more. Results depended on putting the correct amount of toxin in the right place; these were always the same, reliable, and consistent. Alan Scott used this information to unlock the power of botulinum toxin and apply it in a way that accomplished his initial aim.

From Scott's perspective, the advantage of using botulinum toxin in an extraocular muscle was it could be expected to act in a way that was specific, reliable, and longer lasting than anything he had tried so far. But was it safe? After all, it was the most lethal toxin known to man. Drachman had allayed most of those fears with his tips on handling and by explaining precautions. Buoyed by the positivity of what he had heard and the suggestion he contact Dr. Edward Schantz, botulinum toxin went from the bottom of Scott's list to something to at least try.[2]

Alan Scott had read about botulinum toxin and knew it had been used in the laboratory as a blocking agent. But it took Jampolsky's connection with Dr. Ed Maumenee from the Stanford days; and Daniel Drachman, who encouraged Scott and told him about Ed Schantz, to seal the deal. There would be a learning curve with this new agent, but this was a good start.

Scott Obtains the Toxin

It was time for Scott to obtain the toxin and prepare it for use. He contacted Dr. Schantz in April 1972 with a request for the toxin. The response was favorable. The first sample arrived in San Francisco in a few weeks, in a sealed metal container delivered by the US Postal Service. This started a series of events that would have a far-reaching impact.[3]

In 1972, twenty years after the first report by the physiologist Vernon Brooks that botulinum toxin weakened muscle function, Scott had the muscle-weakening agent he had been seeking. In a stroke of good luck, a primate colony had been established at Smith-Kettlewell for work carried out by other scientists studying brain function. When the experiments conducted by the original researchers were completed, the monkeys would be available to Scott's team.

The animals were healthy, their eyes and eye muscles were normal, and they were free! So, the time was right to proceed with the next step in the lab. In Scott's words, "We had constructed a rational [alternative] model to guide strabismus surgery at Smith-Kettlewell. Now was the time to see if it worked." He started by injecting the botulinum toxin he received from Dr. Schantz into the eye muscles of monkeys.

In 2021, Alan Scott reflected on these events and described them this way:

"Daniel Drachman used botulinum toxin to study hind limb [muscle] development in chicks. He injected small amounts in one limb without damaging the embryo elsewhere, just what we needed. Drachman had obtained toxin from [Dr.] Ed Schantz, who had brought his expertise managing toxins from the Army chemical [biological warfare] facility at Fort Detrick to the University of Wisconsin. He generously supplied us with toxin for most of our subsequent experiments, clinical protocols, and early lots of Botox. Botulism epidemics showed that of the seven botulinum toxins, type A created the greatest muscle paralysis, so we chose type A to work with. After we defined potency and effect on mice and cats, I injected the eye muscles of monkeys with toxin. Over the next few days, paralysis of the injected muscles and altered alignment became apparent. The muscle weakness was restricted to the targeted muscle and lasted several weeks. The exciting outcome was altered eye alignment lasting months! There were only a few local side effects and no apparent systemic toxicity.

"We could immediately see the value of botulinum toxin for application in treating strabismus and realized that it would be useful in treating spasmodic forceful closure of the eyelids (blepharospasm) and even other conditions of muscle overactivity. We compiled these results for our first paper describing botulinum toxin muscle injection in a primate. After this, we conducted subsequent studies to assess the stability, dosing, and toxicity of the toxin . . . to formulate it as a drug [we hoped could be safe and effective] for human use. We changed the protein-stabilizing agent from gelatin, an unapproved animal product, to human serum albumin.

"Although the toxin amounts were initially given in nanograms (billionths of a gram) or micrograms (millionths of a gram), we moved quickly to dosing units based on the mouse LD_{50} tests* because we were interested in the biological activity. We had a good idea from our animal usage of the dosage to use in patients and went on to develop a freeze-dried product that was safe in amount and stable over time."

FIRST REPORT

Scott reported this first use of botulinum toxin type A at the annual meeting of the Association for Research in Vision and Ophthalmology (ARVO) in 1973. I knew he had been doing this work and read the paper with interest. Alan was onto something.[4] The ARVO audience that heard his talk, and readers of the journal article, made up of a wide range of researchers and clinicians who were excited by these findings and were eager to keep a close eye on this line of research. The material presented by Scott was in keeping with the mission statement of the organization, which aimed to "advance research worldwide in understanding the visual system and preventing, treating, and curing its disorders."[5]

In this initial paper describing the use of botulinum toxin to weaken eye muscles, published with several coauthors, Scott described promising results with its first-time use. Other agents used included:

- Diisopropyl fluorophosphate (DFP), an agent that had been used extensively in research as a model compound of an acetylcholine inhibitor. Its commercial use was as an insect repellent and it had been considered, but never used, in warfare.
- Alpha-bungarotoxin, a powerful neurotoxin produced by a snake, the krait. This caused paralysis of striated muscles by blocking cholinergic receptors in the neuromuscular junction.

A mouse unit is 7.3×10^{-10} grams, an unwieldy number. When doctors cooperating in the clinical trials first began to receive botulinum toxin type A from Dr. Scott in the 1980s, botulinum toxin amount was measured in nanograms. Investigators were supplied dried toxin and then provided instructions to add normal saline. This dilution in nanograms was psychologically daunting because researchers were dealing with a number nine or ten places to the right of the decimal, or a minus-nine or ten superscript. To some, it seemed entirely too easy to make a mistake and increase the dose a thousand times. Of course, researchers could not really do this because the full contents of the vial were not even close to being dangerous. This reality notwithstanding, it was a great relief to most when the toxin was later provided in biological equivalents so that instead of having dilutions at billionths of a gram, users could have vials containing one hundred biological units. Calculating for a seventy-kilogram human, the LD_{50} would be three thousand units. Since the total of injections per patient at the time were twenty-five to fifty units and not likely to exceed one hundred and later two hundred units, patients were not at risk.

First Injection in a Primate   93

- Alcohol, which in the lab is 95 percent ethanol and 5 percent methanol (drinking it can make you blind). The result from injecting alcohol caused so much redness and reaction in the first monkey it was used only that one time.

Results of injecting the extraocular muscles in monkeys, as reported in the 1973 paper, using these agents, showed that botulinum toxin type A was unequivocally the best, and from that point it was the only agent Scott used for muscle weakening. However, he was cautious in stating that "the chronic clinical relevance of the use of botulinum neurotoxin or other drug injection in the extraocular muscles awaits appropriate human trials."[6]

This initial paper describing results with botulinum toxin contained Scott's carefully worded statement: "Such a pharmacological approach may be used to replace or augment existing methods for surgical treatment for correction of strabismus. The weakening of overacting extraocular muscles . . . and the weakening of the antagonist muscles in paralytic squint both as treatment and in smaller doses to prevent secondary contraction is possible . . . [in addition] extension of this approach to reducing lid retraction in endocrine exophthalmos, reducing blepharospasm and influencing somatic muscle groups responsible for voluntary movement seems entirely feasible."

In this report, Scott delivered a clear statement that he was aware of the effect of the toxin on other muscles, including the large muscles of the limbs and trunk. Expansion of the use of Botox was something he expected from the beginning; when it happened, it was no surprise.

Even though the initial injection of botulinum toxin was limited to extraocular muscles in primates, this research paved the way for use of the toxin in other muscles in humans, including those around the face and neck, and to treat rhytids (wrinkles). Although expanded use of the toxin was not a surprise to Dr. Scott, the extent might have been, especially its use for cosmetic purposes. He was fully aware of the drug's potential. He just was not particularly interested in using the toxin for aesthetics, but he did unselfishly share his experience early on with those who were and offered encouragement.[7] This was noted by those who knew the true history of the development of Botox.[8] This awareness, or recognition, did not always carry over to patients who received cosmetic treatment, proclaiming their own doctor invented Botox. When it came to recognizing the full scope of this drug, Alan Scott was neither naïve nor avaricious. He instead persisted in his targeted focus on the treatment of eye muscles in patients with strabismus.

Initial Success

Success using botulinum toxin, the most lethal toxin known to mankind, resulted in sustained weakening of an eye muscle in a primate and changed eye alignment without harm to the subject—a crowning achievement so far. That success was built on ten years of work in the laboratory. It started with studies that used electromyography of the extraocular muscles, mostly in humans, with advice from experts like Carter Collins and David Robinson that paved the way by demonstrating how each of the extraocular muscles behaved during any movement of the eyes. Then to enable delivery of the toxin to a precise location in the exact dose, the Teflon-coated needle of Scott's design was an important enabler. At the conclusion of an orderly process, a toxin with the right properties was tamed with dilution, and its stability made it safe for injection in a monkey.

Based on results in the monkeys, Scott predicted that weakening an individual eye muscle would be a way to achieve balance that would benefit a patient with strabismus by producing straight or straighter eyes after injection of the appropriate normal or overacting muscle. With these encouraging results from injection of botulinum toxin, further evaluation of this agent was warranted. At this point, Alan Scott and his team at Smith-Kettlewell had completed the second phase of their study. They had corralled a lethal toxin by showing it was both safe and effective for their purposes in the laboratory. In a program where the next hurdle always looms larger, their challenge was to determine if the toxin was safe and effective in a human.

Moving Forward

Scott had been practicing for nearly fifteen years. His family was increasing, his private practice was successful, and his laboratory was producing promising results. Life for him could be compared to the juggler who must keep all the balls in the air, treating each with appropriate care to keep the act in motion. It took an understanding spouse—and Ruth Scott was just that. Alan was able to devote sufficient attention to each aspect of his life and this led to success all around.

Based on the exciting results from the lab, the next step for Scott was to obtain an Investigator New Drug (IND) approval from the Food and Drug Administration (FDA). He needed this authorization before moving on to testing botulinum toxin type A in a human. His first step involved presenting the results of the study so far. They demonstrated the drug was safe in a primate (monkey), and that it did what it was supposed to do. He had assembled compelling evidence that the botulinum toxin injected in an extraocular muscle was both safe and effective. Completing the application would be a breeze and he thought approval for human studies would be granted to him promptly.

However, the rest of the process, according to Scott, was "not so easy. . . . Our application lay on some FDA desk for almost four years! When a colleague . . . moved from Harvard Chief of Ophthalmology to the National Eye Institute in Washington, DC, he kindly put in a word supporting our application and it was approved in a few days."[9]

Thanks to an established working relationship with Dr. Ed Schantz, Scott was confident botulinum toxin would be available to conduct the necessary trials involving human subjects. Back home and working full time at the Wisconsin Food Institute of the University of Wisconsin–Madison, Schantz might have relished being "back in the game." After the initial contact, Schantz "generously supplied toxins," Scott said.

With IND approval in hand, Scott was able to take the next crucial step to advance the status of botulinum toxin type A from a death-dealing poison to a useful drug for humans.

15

First Injection in a Human

Human clinical trials begin.

When someone seeks approval for a new drug to be used in humans, federal laws, enforced through regulating interstate commerce, remain the foundation for a powerful consumer protection policy. This is the backbone of the Food and Drug Administration (FDA). The rules put forth by this agency are clearly defined, and compliance must be unwavering. The safe food and drugs now available are the welcome result of this diligence.[1]

Anyone who seeks approval for a new drug is advised to obtain guidance from the FDA before beginning because the drug approval procedure includes multiphase clinical trials that must be carried out, adhering to a process both demanding and exacting. With his Investigational New Drug (IND) approval in hand, Scott knew the third stage of his own effort would be guided by the strict rules surrounding the official FDA clinical trial protocol. That represented a unique and formidable challenge.

Scott was confident of success and eager to proceed. He had completed extensive studies of the workings of the human extraocular muscles. His initial experiments injecting extraocular muscles in monkeys reported in 1973 were successful.[2] He had found a biological agent that was safe and effective, and he was promised more supplies would be available. Finally, both the Smith-Kettlewell Eye Research Institute and California Pacific Medical Center would remain as sponsors for his research.

With the shift to human subjects, Smith-Kettlewell continued to have a significant role in the research effort. This is where most of the procedures dealing with management of the botulinum toxin in a human would be carried out. California Pacific Medical Center, including facilities and staff, would play an even more important role as human subjects were added to the protocol. Scott anticipated approval, and even encouragement, from his local supporters as he approached the next rung of the ladder of institutional rigor. He was not disappointed. Reaching out to the federal government was different. It was impersonal and represented a big step for an individual researcher. Alan Scott took it in stride.

Smith-Kettlewell had been the main site for the experiments involving botulinum toxin type A injected in the extraocular muscle of primates. Now, phase two of the study was completed. Smith-Kettlewell's oversight with the preparation of toxin for use in a human would be carried out in their facility as well as in certified laboratories and manufacturing facilities used by Scott. These efforts would fulfill requirements of the FDA but were confined to oversight of the drug itself.

With the toxin injected in humans, Scott's initial encounters with these patients was at California Pacific Medical Center under the supervision of the hospital's institutional review board (IRB). This board comprised a panel of scientists and others in the hospital who determined whether the research plan was sound. In this process, patient safety was paramount. According to established practice, "The IRB is concerned with protecting the welfare, rights, and privacy of human subjects. The IRB has the authority to approve, disapprove, monitor, and require modifications in all research activities that fall within its authority as specified by both the federal regulations and institutional policy."[3] In addition to FDA approval that the drug was safe and effective, what type of material (protocol) was submitted to an IRB for evaluation before embarking on a new drug's clinical trial? It turned out to be a lot!

This application required a comprehensive description of the type of subjects who could participate. It also included the schedule of tests and procedures, the medications and dosages to be studied, the length of the study, and the study's objectives. Additional details unique to the investigation that would be key to any decision were also to be included. The IRB made sure the work to be done was acceptable according to their own criteria.

Along with evidence that the research had advanced to the state where it would be prudent to continue, the usual requirements were that participants had given consent and were fully informed of any risks, and that researchers took appropriate steps to protect patients from harm. The process had interdependent components, including the FDA who set the rules and was the final arbiter. Other participants included the researchers who carried out experiments and the patient (subject) who agreed to an intervention that promised but did not guarantee results. Finally, and key to the entire process, was the institution working through its review board, which is the guarantor ensuring measures were in place to keep patients safe and that all work carried out in the study was done according to established guidelines.

Beyond these oversight requirements, Scott had to deal with practical matters; foremost was the need for more people to complete the multitude of tasks that were added. The most pressing issue was compliance with the rules for manufacturing a drug.

In an act of providence, help arrived just in time when Dennis Honeychurch, a former radiopharmacist with the navy, joined the effort. He had experience with manufacturing practices and agreed to play a key role in the manufacture. Moreover, money to support the formation of a new corporation to manufacture the drug was gained when Scott, after a serious talk with Ruth, decided to raise money by mortgaging their house! The Scott's designed and played a significant role in building this house in the sixties and it remained their home for life. In terms of available toxin, Scott was buoyed by the steadfast support of Dr. Edward Schantz, who said he would continue to supply whatever toxin was necessary for future studies.

With FDA's IND approval granted, and California Pacific Medical Center and Smith-Kettlewell onboard, clinical trials for botulinum toxin type A began.[4] At this point, most individuals working on their own, like Alan Scott, would have paused to reflect and wonder if it was all worth it. *Am I up to this? What if I fail, will it be overwhelming? What will it cost?* If any of these questions weighed on Alan Scott's mind, they never surfaced. He proceeded with unflagging zeal and unbridled optimism.

THE TRIALS BEGIN

FDA clinical trials are carried out in three phases that are described as follows.[4] Phase 1 studies are usually conducted with healthy volunteers. The goal at this stage is to *determine what the drug's most frequent side effects are* and, often, how the drug is metabolized and excreted. The number of subjects typically ranges from twenty to eighty.

If Phase 1 studies do not reveal unacceptable toxicity, Phase 2 studies begin. While the emphasis in Phase 1 is on safety, the emphasis in Phase 2 is on effectiveness. This phase aims to obtain preliminary data on whether the drug works in people who have a certain disease or condition. For controlled trials, patients receiving the drug are compared with similar patients receiving a different treatment—usually an inactive substance (placebo) or a different drug. Safety continues to be evaluated, and short-term side effects are studied. Typically, the number of subjects in Phase 2 studies ranges from a few dozen to about three hundred.

At the end of Phase 2, the FDA and sponsors can meet to come to an agreement about how many patients should be included in Phase 3. These studies gather more information about safety and effectiveness, studying different populations and dosages, and using the drug in combination with other drugs. The number of subjects usually ranges from several hundred to about three thousand people.

Scott shared that he had no contact with the FDA during a five-year period in the 1980s, when all three phases of his clinical trials were being conducted. Between 1974 and 1989, in nine of those fifteen years, Alan Scott had no communication with the FDA. He was navigating a demanding course on his own.

Another important time for an investigator or sponsor to meet with the FDA is right before a new drug application is submitted. This is an application for the drug to go on the market, and the relationship does not end there. Certain post-market requirements must be met after the FDA has approved a product for marketing. The FDA uses post-market results of a drug's use to gather additional information about safety, efficacy, and optimal use.

Clinical trials are a part of the drug approval process and can cost in the tens to hundreds of millions of dollars or even billions.[5,6] In Scott's case, the problem was he had a plan but little money. Undaunted, he began the clinical trials and along the way found novel but effective ways to cover the costs while spending a small fraction of the amount traditionally required to complete these studies.

Phase 1 of the clinical trials required only a small number of patients who were closely supervised. This work was done mostly by Scott at California Pacific Medical Center and in his clinic. The first human patient selected for treatment of strabismus using botulinum toxin type A was a twenty-six-year-old man. His left eye deviated outward after surgery performed by another doctor to repair a detached retina. The patient was an otherwise healthy individual. He was informed he was the first human to undergo this form of treatment and that Dr. Scott, based on his own studies, was confident it was safe and that he would not be harmed. It was further explained that this procedure had been done in the laboratory for several years and that it had been deemed safe for use in a human by the Food and Drug Administration, a group that took their responsibility seriously in matters like this. Nonetheless, this must have been something the patient gave considerable thought to before deciding to go ahead. The confidence instilled by Dr. Scott and the competence that he showed must have had a sufficiently positive effect. The patient agreed to the procedure.

Not all the trepidation was felt by the patient. In recalling this event, Scott said, "Despite extensive experience characterizing toxin and injecting many animals, it was still an experience to inject the first human patient in 1978."[7] In another instance, commenting on his feelings at the time of this first injection, the usually laconic researcher admitted to feeling a certain anxiety, not about the technique but because of the human subject.

Scott, according to the dictates of the sponsoring institution, accepted California Pacific Medical Center to be the site as a precautionary measure. For the hospital, there were unknowns, especially for administrators and other personnel responsible for the safety of patients. They were also concerned about liability assumed by the hospital. This led California Pacific Medical Center to require injections be done in a hospital operating room with an anesthesiologist and other emergency personnel available. Another precaution was to keep the patient in the intensive care unit for a specified period.

After injection, the patient remained in the hospital for three days where he would be under close observation, making it possible for him to receive immediate care for resuscitation or breathing management with a ventilator if needed. Later, when several additional patients did well, the requirement for injections done in the hospital was dropped, and injections were done without incident in an office setting.

The dose used for the first subject was small, less than 0.2 billionths of a gram (less than one mouse unit) in keeping with safety guidelines imposed by the FDA.[8] It had no apparent effect on eye alignment or muscle behavior. More importantly, it caused no harm. The drug at this dose was safe. The same dose was used for two more patients—again with no effect and no complications. For the fourth patient, the dosage was increased slightly. A moderate weakening of the muscle and improvement in alignment was noted. With subsequent subjects, the dose was increased until the hoped-for effect was achieved. The trial was underway, the drug was having an effect, and there had been no harm done to any patients.

TECHNIQUE FOR INJECTION

The patient is supine (on the back), on a table in a treatment room, in an outpatient office or clinic. This was determined a safe and convenient practice after several patients received injections done in the hospital. The patient remained dressed in street clothes and the chest was covered with a drape.

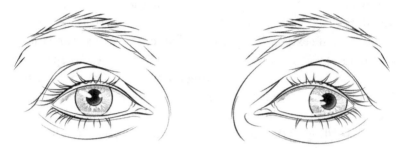

The eyes in this patient are not "straight." The left eye is deviating outward, creating an exotropia. The left lateral rectus (out pulling) muscle must be weakened an appropriate amount to allow the eye to move toward the center, becoming straight or straighter. In this case botulinum toxin will be injected in the left lateral rectus muscle.

Several drops of local anesthetic are placed on the eye to numb the surface layers. They take effect in seconds and no other anesthetic is required.

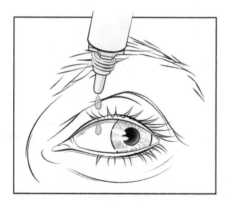

Several drops of local anesthetic are placed on the surface of the eye.

A sound-amplifying device connects the patient with the needle that delivers the toxin. The device creates a sound when exposed to an electrical current. Wires connected the machine to the metal hub of a very fine needle covered with a thin Teflon sheath leaving only the metal at the tip exposed. The electrical current, arising when a nerve stimulates an extraocular muscle, is picked up by the bare-metal tip and carried by a wire through the receiving box grounded at the patient's forehead. Sound from a current entering at the tip of the needle (where it touches muscle) and continuing through this instrument confirms the needle is properly placed at the junction where the nerve activates the muscle.

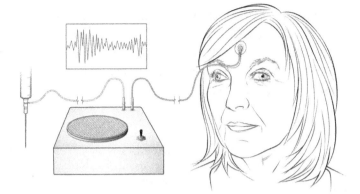

The electromyography recording device connects to the needle hub with one lead and to the patient with another. Both leads should be long enough to accommodate the instrument and provide sufficient access for the operator.

One hundred units of freeze-dried botulinum toxin type A is reconstituted with one or two milliliters of normal saline. Each tenth of a milliliter contained either five or ten units depending on the dilution. After drawing up the dose of toxin intended, plus 0.3 mL with no visible air bubbles, any unseen air bubbles that might be trapped in the needle are eliminated by pointing the needle up and flushing 0.3 mL into a waste container. That same container also collects other disposable equipment used. During these studies, it had been determined that actions such as splashing and pouring of the toxin in a manner like this destabilized the molecules and rendered them harmless.

The dose for the first patient (not employing units) was $.173 \times 10^{-9}$. This small dose, ordered by the FDA, was not expected to have a treatment effect but to look for any adverse reaction. None was observed.[9]

The intended dose of toxin is drawn in the syringe plus sufficient excess to flush out any air in the device.

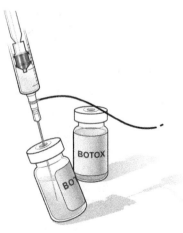

The patient is directed to look to the right, away from the muscle being injected. In this case, the left lateral rectus, the muscle to be injected, was just visible beneath the conjunctiva covering it. Fine-tooth forceps grasp the tissue adjacent to the cornea, stabilizing the eye while the needle punctures the layer covering the muscle.

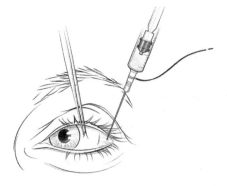

The eye looking away from the muscle to be injected is held in place while the needle is readied.

The needle is then rotated so that the long axis of the needle and syringe align with the muscle. A faint crackling is heard when the needle enters the muscle while the patient continues to look away from the muscle that is to be injected.

The needle enters the muscle, a faint crackling of electrical activity is heard.

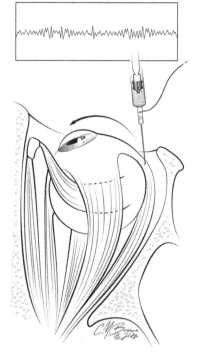

The needle is advanced in the body of the muscle between the globe and the bony wall of the orbit. When the needle reaches the muscle/nerve junction, the crackling sound increases slightly. The patient is then asked to look toward the muscle. When the crackling sound continues to increase, the intended dose is injected, and the needle is removed. If the sound does not increase, the needle is repositioned slightly until the proper location is achieved before injection.

The needle is advanced in the muscle, the patient is asked to look in the direction of the muscle's pull. When the needle tip reaches the site where the nerve enters the muscle and a marked increase in the crackling of electrical activity is heard, the full content of the syringe is injected. The needle is withdrawn immediately.

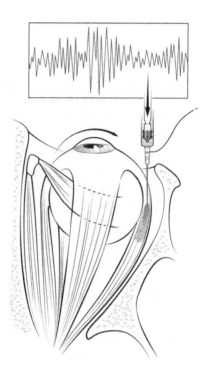

Afterward there might be a slight redness where the needle entered the conjunctiva and there would not be an immediate change in the deviation. It took a few days to a week for the full effect of the toxin to be noted. The change in alignment depended on the strength of the antagonist muscle.

The left eye deviated outward before injection.(above) After the injection, slight redness occurs at the site. The eye moves toward the center in a few days, depending on the weakness of the injected muscle and the pull of its antagonist. (below) A common result in a treatment like this would be a small residual deviation as shown here in the left eye. (Or the eye may be straight or overcorrected and turning in but these results recede with time as the eye frequently drifts toward the pre-injection alignment.) This result could last for months or be permanent, depending on the relative strength of the muscle opposing the treated muscle.

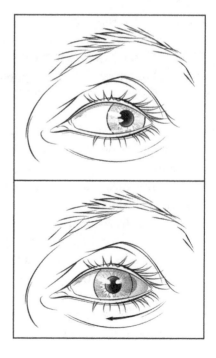

After injection of the toxin, the left lateral rectus pulled out less, but the final position depends on the medial rectus pull against the treated (newly weakened) muscle.

Once the patient was prepared, the procedure took approximately five minutes.

For Alan Scott, the initial in-hospital injection was the culmination of seventeen years of trial and error. It takes amazing dedication and a special type of person to stick with a project like this. "Alan was a smart guy who liked to figure things out," said a student who trained under Scott as the first humans were being treated at the outset of the trials.[10]

When the procedure caused no harm in any patient, except for short-term drooping of the lid, and produced a positive result in the fourth patient who received a slightly increased dose of toxin, Scott continued to treat patients with carefully titrated doses that continued to produce the desired results. Later injections were done safely in an outpatient setting. He made this project the subject of his thesis for acceptance into the American Ophthalmologic Society. In the paper that was published in 1981 and which he delivered at the annual meeting, Scott summarized the work as follows: "One hundred thirty-two doses of botulinum A toxin were injected into forty-two humans. After the proper dose was established, the effect on horizontal strabismus was uniformly beneficial, and the effect lasted up to 411 days since the last injection was documented. The effect in vertical strabismus and lid retraction was beneficial, but less strongly so. No systemic effect or local complications were encountered except for effect on adjacent muscles. The drug appears to be a safe and useful therapy for strabismus."[11]

Scott's choice of words demonstrates both his candor and humility, especially the concluding sentence, when he finished not with a grandiose statement but wrote, "The drug appears safe and useful." This is another example of Alan Scott's penchant for understatement.

He further explained that in the case of a paralyzed muscle, weakening the opposing muscle with an injection of botulinum toxin may have an initial but "incomplete" effect altering alignment but did not last unless the offending underacting muscle (antagonist) was able to regain strength and tone. This meant an untreated muscle must become more effective as it worked against its temporarily toxin-weakened opposite pulling muscle.

Moreover, he explained the most effective use of a botulinum toxin injection was for *concomitant strabismus*, a type of eye misalignment where the muscles of each eye work normally on their own, just not together. Achieving straighter, though not perfectly aligned, eyes after treatment of one or two of these muscles relied on the reflex action of the brain. Better alignment in these cases ultimately depended on the central nervous system fusion mechanism functioning in the brain and benefiting from the toxin's effect. This kind of unpretentious and factual reporting made it easy to believe what was being said by this researcher. Scott's brutal honesty about the limitations of his new treatment was fair warning for potential users. And it was later confirmed by the relatively low number of patients with strabismus who were eventually treated with Botox. According to Scott, the number was about 3 percent.[12]

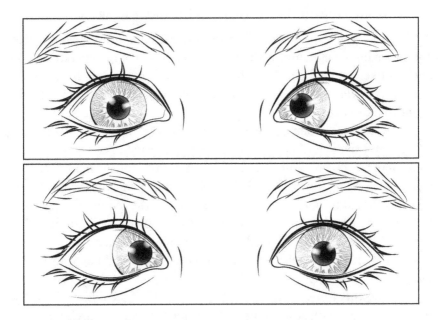

Concomitant strabismus. (above) With the right eye fixing, the left eye is turned in. (below) With the left eye fixing, the right eye is turned in. Both eyes have full rotation and look "straight" with the other eye covered.

In a case of acute muscle palsy that could recover on its own, weakening the opposite muscle with botulinum toxin type A allowed the affected muscle to regain strength sooner in the absence of pull from the opposing muscle. This can be likened to using a cast to stabilize an arm while a broken bone heals or patching a good eye to force the other eye to gain strength in cases of amblyopia, when vision is lost in an eye from disuse or suppression. Using botulinum toxin type A to weaken the muscle can be thought of as a temporary measure in a condition that can improve if given a chance.

Now that Scott had demonstrated the drug was safe and effective for treatment in a human, he decided to move on to the next stage with Phase

2 and 3 trials that would make it possible for botulinum toxin type A to be available for use by hundreds of clinical investigators following Food and Drug Administration (FDA) guidelines. Alan Scott enlisted clinical investigators and introduced them to the techniques he had developed in Phase 1. He expected to be working closely with the FDA, but as the trial progressed, there was little contact. Scott and his team were on their own.

Moving On after the Initial Report

At this time, the "vibes" Scott felt from the FDA about business practices and procedures made him realize he needed to make his operation more businesslike. So, he formed Oculinum Inc. The name came from joining the words *ocular* and *alignment* and became a descriptive term that also sounded like a drug name.

Between 1981, when his thesis was published, approval of the drug in 1989, and the sale of Oculinum to Allergan in 1991, Alan Scott and his team were busy with clinical trials, organizing a company, manufacturing a drug, and trying (unsuccessfully) to sell the whole operation to a suitable pharmaceutical company willing to take it over. The regulations put forth by the FDA, when it came to the myriad tasks involved, were daunting. They called for action with results that demanded a structure and organization that only an established company could provide. Alan Scott faced a monumental challenge.

During this time, Scott concentrated on what he could do best, like treating patients with strabismus and dystonia or spastic muscles that represented expanded indications, while he trained new colleagues in the use of botulinum toxin type A to prepare them to become clinical researchers.

As his work treating patients with the toxin progressed, Scott continued to share unselfishly what he was learning. One of those with whom he shared data was a young ophthalmologist who visited Scott. She would become the person to launch Botox for cosmetic use, gaining approval in Canada in 2001. It was approved in the United States a year later.

16

Joining the Team

Becoming part of the clinical research team in 1982.

Encouraged by success with botulinum toxin to treat not only strabismus but also a wide range of other dystonias and muscle-based maladies, it became evident to Alan Scott that he was onto something that could be used by many. Some conditions that had been treated effectively with the toxin by others in the trial were not only unexpected, but they were also "off the chart." These included conditions like relief of sweaty palms, focal dystonia of the fingers, overactive bladder, laryngeal spasm, and grinding teeth. Botulinum toxin type A was effective in treating these conditions, and it caused no unwanted side effects—that was good to know.

Although he would have been justified in seeking approval of the drug for an array of uses, Scott chose a safer course. He relied on results backed largely by his own data and which could be submitted with confidence to the Food and Drug Administration (FDA). The data were limited to the use of the toxin in eye muscles and dystonias, mostly around the head and neck. Collection of these manageable data became the focus of Scott's efforts. Though he knew the drug had potential for wider use, holding to a narrow list of indications had the advantage of making it easier for the FDA to act quickly. In doing so, they placed Oculinum in the special category of orphan drugs. This designation meant that although it had important use, Oculinum served a small market that limited the amount of money the drug could make. In this case, the term *orphan* simply meant the drug needed help.

This strategy had several advantages, including seven years of exclusivity after approval. Later, off-label uses of the drug that had been proven safe would be the better way to expand use. Despite travail that lay ahead, Alan

Scott had no second thoughts, nor was he entertaining any hesitancy in following a course that would soon result in him becoming a de facto drug manufacturer with Oculinum Inc.

Scott summed up his experiences: "After initial success in strabismus, physicians beyond ophthalmology became interested in using toxin for use in neurology, GI conditions, cerebral palsy, excessive sweating and more. We wound up running an open trial with over two hundred investigators who at the peak were using more than 10,000 vials annually."[1]

I JOIN THE CLINICAL TRIALS

I completed initial training in ophthalmology at Indiana University in 1966 and spent a year in fellowship at Johns Hopkins before returning to the faculty at Indiana University in 1967. This time was stretched by two years because I was drafted halfway through the first year of my residency. I served as a general medical officer in the US Army Medical Corps in Minneapolis. While there, and due to a quirk in rules of the doctor draft, I had the opportunity to work on weekday afternoons and Saturdays in an ophthalmology office—where I learned a lot. This experience in a private general ophthalmology setting, working with Dr. Malcolm A. McCannel, included seeing the grandchildren of Franklin Roosevelt. This two-year experience proved to be the stimulus for my selecting a career in academic medicine, a decision I never regretted.

During my fellowship year, I had my initiation to crossed eyes in a monkey. It happened while I was studying under Gunter K. von Noorden. Since to the best of our knowledge there were no naturally occurring cross-eyed monkeys, I was tasked with making a monkey cross-eyed as part of Dr. von Noorden's experiments studying visual development in a primate. There were no readily available guidelines for doing this in the lab. I did know it took more than simply shifting the position of a muscle that was otherwise normal and able to contract. When others had tried this after a few days, the monkey's eye alignment returned to normal. Instead, my approach was to anchor the eyeball to the wall of the orbit so it could not move. This worked, and the monkey was suitable for purposes of the experiment my mentor was conducting. The job would have been easier with some of Scott's botulinum toxin, but that would not be available for another decade![2]

I knew Alan Scott through our professional involvement with the diagnosis and treatment of patients with strabismus and through our activity with the International Strabismological Association. In the 1970s, only a small number limited their practice to the new sub-specialty of pediatric ophthalmology and strabismus. Like him, I was involved in studying the workings of the extraocular muscles, both normal and defective, and how to treat those not functioning as they should. Scott's work with botulinum toxin was important, and I followed it closely.

Alan Scott and I, along with a small group of young ophthalmologists led by a few of our teachers, were part of a movement that made a new subspecialty official: pediatric ophthalmology and strabismus. There were some "old timers and part-timers" leading the group, but the vibrant new growth was young doctors like us, who enjoyed professional kinship even while working in our own areas at a distance. At that time, before the technology we take for granted today, we connected by letter and phone, and our personal contacts took place mostly at professional meetings.

After Scott described the first successful use of botulinum toxin in a human, he continued working mostly in his own clinic and laboratory. We had the opportunity to discuss his work in 1982 at the meeting of the International Strabismological Association held in Asilomar, California. Asilomar was just north of Pebble Beach on Monterey Bay, virtually in his backyard. After learning more about what Alan was doing, we agreed I would visit his clinic in a few months to learn about the project firsthand. By that time, I had known Alan professionally for nearly ten years and was always impressed with his honesty and skill and would now appreciate his openness and sharing.

I arrived in San Francisco for the meeting accompanied by my partner in practice at Indiana University School of Medicine, Daryel Ellis. Alan showed us his lab, clinic, and operating room in San Francisco and explained how he used electromyography. He demonstrated his injection technique on an infant and impressed us with his skill as he did it with ease. This took place in what could be best characterized as a bare-bones but adequate outpatient environment—no fluff! We immediately accepted his offer for us to become participants in the open clinical trial of botulinum toxin.

We were among the early group of clinical investigators meeting with Alan individually as experienced and familiar colleagues. Our orientation comprised observation and discussion over two days. Scott's admonition was to use the drug as we saw fit based on our experience and the needs of our patients. By doing this we were assured that the drug was safe and predictable, but its potential had not yet been tapped. However, it was implied that our first efforts would be to test its use in our patients being treated for strabismus.

We were given no specific reporting requirements but urged to tell him about any complications our patients experienced. Later in the trials, as more investigators were recruited, many of whom he would be meeting for the first time, Scott's protocol stiffened. He accepted formal applications and set up regular training sessions in groups of a dozen. In a classroom setting, he would describe the drug and its uses and demonstrate techniques and equipment needed. Some of this he made available at an affordable price. Important in these sessions was explaining a detailed reporting process describing the patients treated, the results of treatment, and the lot number of medicine used. These data were sent to Scott, who compiled them as part of the study. The most important contribution of these data related to side effects and complications, both of which were exceedingly rare (and reassuring!).

On returning to our clinic in Indianapolis, where I was head of the Section of Pediatric Ophthalmology and a newly minted professor, we purchased equipment necessary for electromyography, including the Scott-designed, Teflon-coated needles. We set aside a devoted area in the department for this work and looked forward to receiving the first vials of botulinum toxin type A.

Our initial patients were treated at Indiana University Hospital, at James Whitcomb Riley Hospital for Children, and in the ophthalmology outpatient clinic in the Rotary Building. At first, we used the toxin in strabismus cases to weaken the antagonist of a paralyzed or severely underacting muscle that was also receiving surgical treatment, including shortening and, in some cases, with transfer of the action of adjacent muscles. We had no complications with the treatments and could see results that suggested there could be a use for this technique. Our conclusion was to use this in our practice during the trial. It would support and not replace the surgical procedures we were already using.

Soon, in the spirit of this being an open trial, which meant we could use the toxin in any way we saw fit, our use evolved. Adult patients with different ailments started to show up. They suffered from the effects of uncontrolled contraction of their facial muscles (dystonia) and the uncontrolled forceful closure of the lids (blepharospasm). These conditions were embarrassing for the individual, and they interfered with everyday activities.

Most important with these patients, botulinum toxin type A was the only treatment we had available that could help them. It was a godsend.

The uncontrolled muscle contractions experienced by these patients were not only disruptive in social contact; in severe cases they made it impossible for a person to drive a car safely or even walk across a street unaided. Many of these patients had uncontrolled grimacing that was both unpleasant and socially limiting. They needed help, and botulinum toxin type A seemed to be the answer.

Although we treated some adults, children with any type of eye problem made up the bulk of our practice. They always came with a parent or two and maybe a sibling. For everybody's comfort and well-being, we established a separate area for the adult patients we treated in our regular Oculinum clinic. Soon we were seeing hundreds of patients. They returned every three to five months for regular injections. Each session included about a dozen patients seen in the adult section of the department. We assigned a technician to oversee the management of these clinics. The botulinum toxin was initially provided free by Dr. Scott. Later he suggested we donate twenty-five dollars, then forty dollars, for a one-hundred-unit vial to cover Scott's ever-escalating costs. The toxin continued to be offered to our patients at no charge, as were the treatments that were not covered by Medicare or most other insurance plans. Our clinic functioned flawlessly, and soon we were treating a dozen patients at each clinic session.

In 1985, a fifty-five-year-old woman presented at the clinic with a special problem—or rather, problems! She had suffered a stroke and was in a wheelchair. The left side of her face and body were paralyzed. Because of extensive damage from corneal exposure and infection, the left eye was blind. Her potentially "good" right eye had uncontrolled movement in every direction because of nerve damage to the muscles caused by her stroke. Her right eye had the potential to see normally, but the constant movement kept her from watching TV or reading. When she tried to look at the world, she saw images that appeared jumbled and confused. She was desperately searching for help.[3] We had nothing to offer her using our standard treatments. What about botulinum toxin?

Earlier we had tried treating another patient with blurred vision from uncontrolled eye movement. In her case, we started by injecting individual muscles around one eye. That failed. Next, I injected twenty-five units of the toxin in the orbit behind the right eye. This turned out to be the first time this had been done in a human. It was done in the operating room as a precaution, and there were no problems. The next day the treated eye was moving less, and vision had improved. The patient returned to the care of her doctor, and we had no further contact. The woman was in poor health from multiple causes and we heard nothing further from her physician.

Based on these promising but inconclusive results, we offered this second patient a retrobulbar injection to treat her remaining sighted eye. This woman, despite her many problems, had a heart, lungs, and cognitive brain that were all functioning well. She also possessed a strong will to get on with her life as best as she could.

We did the procedure in the outpatient clinic after explaining that the drug was in the clinical trial phase and not yet approved. We added the caveat that to the best of our knowledge, this toxin had never been injected behind the eye except by us, and then only once without long-term follow-up. This news did not deter the patient. She simply said, "The way I am now, what do I have to lose?"

A day after the injection, her eye was stable with only limited voluntary movement. Her vision looking straight ahead was excellent. The reduced side gaze did not bother her. Her pupil was dilated. This was of no consequence, just an expected response to the botulinum toxin. The good news was her uncorrected vision in the distance was normal. More important, objects she saw remained still and were seen clearly. This provided her with vision suitable for watching TV comfortably, and she could read small print using her reading glasses.

This was a win for the patient and for botulinum toxin. The improved level of acuity experienced by this woman persisted for several months. After this, unwanted eye movements returned, and her vision gradually worsened. The patient returned when she decided another injection was needed. The routine continued for several years, always with a good result. During this time, she developed no immunity to the drug—more good news. Eventually, more than a dozen patients were treated by us successfully this way, and others have employed this technique.

This previously untried and likely unthought-of use of botulinum toxin was made possible by Alan Scott launching an open clinical trial. The drug being tested had a wide margin of safety, had a specific localized and dose-related effect on the nerve-muscle connection, and had not to date demonstrated unacceptable side effects in either his lab or clinic. The drug's range of use was limited only by how far each investigator was willing to push the envelope. The good sense and willingness to explore new options were carried out successfully by a wide range of specialists to meet their patients' unique needs while exploring the options for the versatile drug.

Throughout the trial we received vials with one hundred units of Oculinum. (Scott had renamed botulinum toxin since forming his corporation.) We submitted voluntary donations in the amounts that were suggested in a timely manner. There were no demands, and we never received a bill or a reminder. We received no information about how to best use the toxin other than instruction about how to reconstitute the dried toxin with normal saline. We were free to use Oculinum as we chose if we made it clear to subjects that we were giving them an experimental drug. I can remember no case where a person declined treatment.

After approximately a year, our regular patient load settled into a routine. Twice a month we saw adult patients, mostly seniors with dystonia primarily involving the face and neck. We maintained a regular chart for each patient as part of their clinical record, as we did for all patients. We recorded diagnosis, treatment provided, and results of treatment and would have included complications we encountered, but our patients had none that were significant. Patients were pleased with the results and returned faithfully at intervals when the effects of the drug began to wear off. We were especially heartened to hear stories from grateful patients who reported their lives had been "given back."

In January 1986, our clinic received a call from a woman who told us her husband was able to drive to Florida for the first time in years because the treatment had allowed him to keep his eyes open. This was something that had been impossible before the treatment. Then, after a pause, she said her husband died a few weeks after they arrived in Florida, but she hastened to add that his death was from a different cause. She did finish this bittersweet encounter saying her husband died a happy man. We had satisfied part of his bucket list.

We kept records of our results using botulinum toxin in the laboratory and the clinic and reported them in medical journals and in a textbook. At no time during these studies did we receive any advance information from Scott about results other than those that appeared in medical journals or were reported at meetings. We were told we would be made aware of any significant complications and notices of changes in the protocol if that became necessary. The trials proceeded smoothly, and we received no such directives.

The open clinical trial of botulinum toxin continued for nearly a decade. Soon our use of the toxin to treat patients became just another way to help people who came to us with a need. We had confidence in the drug and had no reservations about its use. It was as much a part of our treatment plan as any approved drug we employed. Our Oculinum clinic continued to provide the drug free and charged little, if anything, for the examinations or follow-up treatment. The clinic operated at close to a break-even level. Our patients were exceedingly happy with the results of treatment, and so were we.

The scales continued to weigh heavily in favor of the drug, and both we and our patients would have been at a loss without it. Of note, this was the only clinic in our department that was named for the single drug it dispensed. I continued to use that name until I retired in 2001. It could have been called Botox in the last ten years we used the drug because that was its name after Allergan purchased Oculinum. We eventually made some adjustments to at least cover the cost of the Botox, but it was hard for us to give up the name Oculinum.

17

Manufacturing Begins

Hundreds of researchers, thousands of patients, and now a corporation.

To supply the growing number of investigators participating in the study with toxin and to comply with the Food and Drug Administration's (FDA's) rule that a biologic agent, a living substance, must be processed by a regular pharmaceutical manufacturing facility, Scott realized there was an urgent need to increase the production of Oculinum. It was time for the project to be put on a business footing.[1]

By now, a sober evaluation of where botulinum toxin type A / Oculinum was headed made it clear that this drug would reach a market beyond what had been envisioned at the start. Acting on this, Scott contacted several established pharmaceutical companies, eight in all, and offered to sell his company, Oculinum. All declined. They had good reason.

The market for this drug for the treatment of strabismus, as intended by Scott, was small. After adding treatment of dystonia in facial and neck muscles as indications for use of the drug, it could be expected to bring in only around $10 million. This was not a big number to a pharmaceutical company. Other disincentives for a prospective buyer were that botulinum toxin was the most lethal toxin known. Moreover, it had no patent protection. Most who knew about botulinum toxin associated it with sickness, or even death, from eating tainted food or from using a dirty needle. Oculinum was not considered a drug worth purchasing for manufacture and sale.

In some ways, Scott was a "victim" of the success of his project. Based on the initial positive results recorded with the first use of the toxin in humans, coupled with rapidly expanding open clinical trials, he was faced with the need to make important decisions for the project to move ahead. This was how he described the challenges he faced:

"It became obvious that we needed to increase our manufacturing capability. This needed to be done even though my primary interest was in research and not in developing a product. Our lab had a patent policy under which we declared items or processes of possible patentability. But the lawyers told us that our 1973 paper had disclosed how the toxin works thus precluding a later patent even though that 1973 paper was years before demonstration of clinical effectiveness. We did not have a patent now and it would never be attainable by anyone. Without one, no 'pharma' company would take over manufacture. So, I took out a loan on my home and formed a corporation, Oculinum Inc., to manage this project."[2]

Continuing, Alan Scott told of a chance event that created forward momentum for the project. "Good fortune brought Dennis Honeychurch to oversee product development in 1983. Dennis had experience with good manufacturing practices (GMP) in his work as a radiopharmacist with the Navy. (A radiopharmacist formulates and distributes medicine with radioactive compounds and, in doing so, must follow strict medical and government guidelines.) We needed the project licensed and [this meant] an establishment license issued by the Food and Drug Administration (FDA) Center for Biologics. This is typically issued to large corporations [but in this case it was necessary for us to act like one]. The project was moved out of the research facility and into a more suitable location in Berkeley, across the street from the animal testing facility."

Scott continued by sharing this report from Dennis Honeychurch, who described his role after 1983 when the manufacture of Oculinum began:[3]

"My involvement started in 1983. Alan had established the safety and efficacy but lacked the license to move [the toxin] out of [investigational new drug] IND status to an approved biological status. We needed a product and establishment license issued by the FDA Center for biologics, typically issued to large corporations under single management. The drug manufacture and testing had to be moved out of the research facility. We did not have the funds or expertise to establish a manufacturing and testing operation, and big pharma wanted to keep their distance.

"The licensing would be creative, and we would need to use outside contractors. Our staff would perform most operations, and even those operations that were contracted out would require them to be present. At first, we started with six people working part time, and when the application was filed, we had a staff of eight mostly full time. The first step was creation of a manual to cover good manufacturing practices and quality assurance. This would cover standard operating procedures, quality control, and include all aspects of the process. In the end we were north of one hundred procedures. Our limiting factor was funds to carry out this program.

"Finding a manufacturing facility to take on the toxin was a dead end until we came up with a manufacturer in Albuquerque, whose only product was water for injection. Alan and I made our first trip to Albuquerque and came away disappointed. We both gowned up, entered a clean room, and prepared a small batch in a laminar flow hood. The batch was handed off to their personnel, and we stayed to observe the rest of the process. This first run did not go well, because the automated filling machine broke numerous vials. Soon after, the process was moved to a class one hundred clean room, and filling was done by hand. Their staff became very efficient at filling and setting stoppers in place on batches of ten thousand vials. Alan and I would continue the trip to formulate and observe, and I often would travel alone and have one of their staff with me in the clean room to check off the master batch record used for compounding. The process called for the vials to be flash frozen and then dried under vacuum. Unlabeled vials were packaged with dry ice and shipped back to San Francisco.

"All testing, storage, and shipping was moved out of the research facility to a building in Berkeley located across the street from an animal testing facility. The animal facility had procedures and documentation in place to meet FDA requirements. This would allow us to comply with the participation portion for licensing. For example, after preparing doses for potency, safety/identity, staff would cross the street and inject the mice [for assay—an experimental method for assessing the presence, localization, or biological activity and strength of a living substance]. Our new facility provided the space needed for the numerous product-testing procedures, labeling, storage, shipping, and office space.

"Here again, the limited budget forced us to be creative. We had a laminar flow hood to perform sterility testing. We needed a clean space with positive pressure to place the hood. Alan and I built this room during a weekend utilizing the air from outside the room to supply the hood in an area with positive pressure. Since our product was dried under vacuum, we needed to validate the process. The final product had only 1.4 milligrams of albumen and sodium chloride, and we had to test down to the microgram range. We could not afford the instrument the FDA used. We ended up connecting several vials with tubing, applied heat, then swept them with dry nitrogen in an inexpensive instrument which could read amounts of moisture to the micrograms."

Alan Scott added his perspective: "The first step toward licensing was to create a document to cover the GMP (good medical practices) and quality assurance, which in total amounted to more than one hundred procedures. FDA allowed us to contract out some of the manufacturing steps to a facility in Albuquerque, New Mexico, provided one of our staff was present during the process. Dennis or I would go up and enter the clean room used for compounding. We were both immunized against the effect of the toxin and, as such, would make the first two critical dilutions. This created diluted toxin that was now safe for the technicians to handle. While we went skiing at Taos, the technicians produced batches of ten thousand vials, which were packed with dry ice and shipped by air back to San Francisco. We were required to declare the dry ice as a hazardous item, but botulinum toxin was exempt.

"In the early days, we asked for donations of twenty-five dollars for each vial of botulinum toxin Type A we sent out to other investigators. The money went to Smith-Kettlewell to pay for our research studies. After that, we hired additional personnel to help with the testing of multiple batches, and the clinical data and statistics on hundreds of cases. We later raised the request for the donation to forty dollars per vial.

"In 1987, we had to stop production as neither the board at Smith-Kettlewell nor the insurers wanted the risk of us distributing toxin for humans. By then, hundreds of patients with blepharospasm, torticollis, spasmodic dysphonia, and so on were clinically dependent on the toxin. They were extremely upset and sent the FDA an avalanche of letters, which caused the FDA to wake up and get actively involved. We were off their radar and had not been visited for five years."

Data from the Clinical Trials

Much of the information I collected for this book, about the years of data collection and trial studies, was acquired during two meetings with Alan Scott in 2021 via Zoom. During our interview sessions, Alan sat comfortably at his desk. Over his left shoulder stood a three-drawer metal file cabinet next to a stout brick wall. All of the drawers were open different amounts and in no purposeful manner displaying an orderly array of documents. On Dr. Scott's right, I surmised, was a bookcase. When a subject came up that was appropriate for fact-checking, Alan would reach in that direction but then retreat his arm and conjure a memory to produce an answer. The papers stayed in the file drawer and the books, for the most part, on their shelves. When we spoke, I was responsible for accurately recording the words of the person who was *there* and *lived* these events told as he remembered them.

The value of the drug was that it worked well and was both safe and reliable. In the beginning, especially for those of us providing the treatment, the fact that the drug wore off in time was reassuring. In cases where the patient had a carryover effect or an unintended spread, we knew it would be transient and revert to the pre-injection state, but that rarely happened.

Despite the monumental disparity between an individual researcher and a giant corporation, the results achieved with this drug approval process for botulinum toxin were the same. The drug was approved, and after more than thirty years of use since that approval, it has proved both safe and effective, with hundreds of millions of units being used and indications for new uses only increasing.

The Drug Is Approved

Oculinum (botulinum toxin type A) was licensed by the FDA on December 29, 1989, for the treatment of strabismus and blepharospasm associated with dystonias in patients twelve years of age and older. About the exclusion of patients under twelve years of age, Scott lamented, "A pediatric ophthalmology consultant to the FDA recommended they disallow usage for children, even though we had supporting data for over eight hundred pediatric cases. It was just a mistake on my part to let this pass, as childhood strabismus treatment with Botox soon became widespread, but only outside the USA." (I suspect Alan knew the name of that person. When I asked, he waved off my question saying, "Let that pass.")

Allergan had a distribution agreement with Oculinum Inc. beginning after the FDA's approval, and the pharmaceutical company acquired Oculinum outright a little over a year later in 1991 and renamed it Botox.

As Scott predicted, Botox has become a major pharmaceutical drug that has proved useful for dozens of conditions in which blocking abnormal nerve conduction to striated muscle is effective in relieving symptoms. Today just over half of Botox goes to these medical conditions, and the rest is used for cosmetics.[4]

When Scott sold Oculinum to Allergan, he recouped his development costs and rewarded Dr. Edward Schantz for the toxin he had supplied for more than twenty years. The money that remained was little more than a token when it came to reimbursing Scott for the thirty years, beginning in 1961, spent working in the laboratory. He earned a living practicing medicine and did it well. But for Scott, there was more. To derive full benefit from his professional life, he needed to experience the satisfaction of finding answers based on his own research. This quest ended only when his life did. The fruits of his studies were an essential part of medicine for Alan Scott. Never in it solely for the money or fame, he established a goal, worked to achieve it, and as a result gained success and satisfaction. That was all he sought.

At the time he sold Oculinum to Allergan, Scott was aware of its wider use but remained focused on the treatment of strabismus and facial dystonia. He did not take a stand against what he knew was an unreasonable restriction on the part of the FDA limiting approval to patients twelve years and older, nor is there evidence he pointed out to the buyer the many other medical uses that had been uncovered, indications that would make the drug more valuable, commanding a higher sale price. Why Scott failed to take advantage of these opportunities was never explained beyond this self-assertion: "I was a lousy businessman."

ALLERGAN

Allergan pharmaceutical remains the producer of Botox, although a great deal has happened to the company in the last thirty years. Soon after the purchase, Allergan, seeing the end in sight for the 79-11 culture prepared by Ed Schantz shortly after Scott carried out the first injection of the toxin in a human, created a new culture. It is produced by them in their own plants that include a dedicated facility in Westport, Ireland. Allergan later withstood a hostile takeover when it was purchased, and some say rescued, by a smaller company, Actavis, that retained the name Allergan. After a brief period, the new Allergan was purchased by Abbott Laboratories, which then spun off ABBVIE as the home for its pharmaceutical products. Through all of this, the venerable name of Allergan persists.

MOVING ON WITH NEW IDEAS

Scott talked about life after Oculinum: "Smith-Kettlewell began to contract in size in about [the year] 2000, with the departure of investigators and closure of its major research facility. Those of us still interested in eye muscle function and strabismus treatment developed the nonprofit Strabismus Research Foundation (SRF) to continue work in San Francisco on those topics. Injections of eye muscles with the local anesthetic bupivacaine to treat strabismus is the first major outcome from SRF. Two hundred and forty clinical cases have shown adding bupivacaine to be more powerful than Botox alone. With the combination of both drugs—Botox in the stronger, overacting muscle and bupivacaine in the weaker, underacting muscles— large deviations can be corrected. This technique creates alignment now shown to last longer providing results fully comparable to surgical correction."[5]

The story of Botox is only growing. And more is being said about the drug Alan Scott developed while working as both the brains and the brawn of this project. Most of the latest news about Botox deals with the reason *Time* magazine displayed Botox on its cover as a Swiss army knife for medicine.[6]

18

Marketing and Selling a New Drug

Once a drug is determined by the Food and Drug Administration to be both safe and effective, it is time for somebody to try and sell it.

"I did what I did because I liked it. If making money had been my goal, there would have been better ways to go."

—*Alan Scott*

Anticipation of market expansion for botulinum toxin no doubt made it possible for Scott to finally complete the sale of the drug to Allergan in 1991 for a reported $9 million. This was both a bargain price for Allergan and a financial respite for Scott. With the Food and Drug Administration's (FDA's) approval of Oculinum, he had accomplished his primary goal, which was not to make lots of money but, in his own words, "figure out some interesting things." He did! In the process, he had mortgaged his home, based on confidence that the eventual sale of Oculinum would allow him to recoup his expenses. The offer from Allergan was enough to put things right with obligations he had to an underpaid staff and a generous and unselfish benefactor who supplied the toxin.

From a vantage of thirty years after the sale, buying Oculinum was more like a steal for Allergan! They paid Alan Scott $9 million for a drug that now sells in the billions, and it would have cost the company hundreds of millions if they had done the development themselves. Even with reason to believe the market would grow, the purchaser must have been overjoyed at the unanticipated bonanza when the full potential of the drug was realized based on off-label use for medical indications and its approval for cosmetic use in both Canada and the United States at the start of the new millennium. Or was Allergan always confident this would happen?

Scott summed it up this way: "I am not sure if we had all the fun and Allergan got all the money, but it was something like that."[1]

Though disclosure in 1973 eliminated any chance of obtaining a patent for the drug, Allergan obtained a valuable trade secret for production of botulinum toxin type A. This provided the new owner a certain level of protection. Though less than a patent, the sanctity of a trade secret can be upheld in legal action. Trade secrets can be violated when employees break confidentiality or when rivals use unlawful means to obtain confidential information. This protection was upheld recently in court, favoring the makers of Botox over a rival.[2]

Trade secrets have no expiration date. They last if the information is kept secret. This could be in perpetuity, as in the case of the famous Coca-Cola formula. Also, competition can be thwarted when the thing is just darn hard to make, as in the case of the world's deadliest toxin. Edward Schantz had shared the toxin widely with researchers but retained the culture. By 1990 it was being produced in the United Kingdom as Dysport. This could be competition, but that was part of life in the industry.

Though Alan Scott's aim was to find a safe and effective alternative to surgery for the treatment of strabismus, it was impossible to ignore the fact that botulinum toxin type A could affect the action of other striated muscles. Moreover, this ubiquitous neurotransmitter affected other bodily functions like sweating and pain, as it acted in a way not fully understood. He had regularly invited specialists in a variety of fields to his clinic in San Francisco, and most of them left eager to find new ways to use the drug to treat the special needs of the patients they served. Scott did not hold back. He shared widely.

In his own field of interest, strabismus, Scott studied the actions of the extraocular muscles in exquisite detail before injecting the toxin in a primate—as an artist might when seeking a precise alteration to obtain a specific effect. The brain that receives the images from the two eyes is guided by these muscles that must provide perfect alignment necessary to achieve normal binocular vision. In Scott's plan, an ideal role for botulinum toxin was for it to recalibrate extraocular muscle action in an infant with concomitant strabismus—"born" with crossed eyes. This could give the brain a second chance to lock in perfect alignment, producing straight eyes. This would take one or two injections. Botox treatment in children with strabismus, including those with early onset, commonly results in a residual deviation of four degrees, not quite straight. This is obtained in just over half with infants under a year achieving better results. These results notwithstanding, most prefer traditional surgery.

Studies comparing Botox with surgery in children of all ages with concomitant strabismus have shown promise, especially in smaller angles, but results have not been conclusive. Further prospective studies with random assignment have been suggested and would likely provide useful information.[3]

After the sale of Oculinum, Scott began to use it in combination with bupivacaine to increase strength in the weaker muscle. He reported excellent results with this technique, but it has yet to achieve widespread use. Elective use for cosmetic indications and treatment for a long list of medical conditions employed in a dozen specialties led by neurology are likely to be the drivers of the Botox market.

Strabismus treatment currently accounts for as little as 1 percent of the Botox used! This is not due to indifference or opposition on the part of physicians. Practical reasons why Botox is not more widely used for strabismus are that treatment with it must be repeated in many cases and it fails to produce better results than surgery. Moreover, there is a "learning curve" to obtain the skill required to deliver the drug safely and effectively. Botox is favored by some for treatment of concomitant strabismus in infants (congenital esotropia), and it does have an additive effect when used in conjunction with some surgical procedures. Botox has been employed successfully in selected cases of acute extraocular muscle weakness and for *oscillopsia*, but the number of patients needing this care is small. Alan Scott discovered the tool and others found a use for it.

While validation of the botulinum toxin was achieved with eye muscle experiments done in a human, success depended on how this valuable information was employed widely for other purposes. The genius of Alan Scott, whose own interest was focused on a narrow scope for treatment, was that he was willing to recognize the wider application of botulinum as he encouraged others. He put no limits on clinical investigators, nor discouraged those who were willing to try something new. But for himself, he stayed the course when it came to remaining true to his original intent, and that centered on strabismus. It continued so with his use of bupivacaine for enhancement of Botox's effect.

Alan Scott's failure to have an agent with him at the sale of Oculinum is validation of his own opinion about his lack of business acumen. A comparable situation with a different outcome is that of the young nephrologists who were part of the development team for Gatorade in the 1960s. When they sold the rights for this drink to Stokely-Van Camp, an Indianapolis company best known for its canned beans, they were represented by an attorney. The result was an agreement that has so far totaled more than $1 billion in royalties. This colored and flavored hydration fluid, now produced by a subsidiary of PepsiCo Inc., sold more than $6.25 billion in 2022.

A Close Call for Allergan

By 2015, Botox was a high-flying drug with strong brand recognition. It led the world market. Botox also had its own unique "protection." It is a biologic that demands special skills to produce. The overall recipe is known, but the fine points carried out in the process of developing and maintaining the culture are closely held trade secrets. An aggressive Canadian pharmaceutical company that was a "takeover" specialist and not interested in developing their own drug decided Allergan was a ripe target for acquisition. This resulted in a narrow escape caused by a company that had started a maelstrom in the high-stakes drug arena.

If the acquisition by Valeant Pharmaceutical had been successful, Botox—which sold close to half of the botulinum toxin used worldwide—could have seen prices skyrocket. Valeant Pharmaceutical had raised the monthly dosage price of Syprine, a lifesaving drug that treats a rare liver condition known as Wilson's disease, to $21,267 per month in 2015, from $652 just five years earlier.[3] This new pricing meant it would cost a patient nearly a quarter of a million dollars a year for maintenance—to stay alive! Merck Pharmaceutical developed the drug earlier and sold it for one dollar a pill to treat this rare disease, which can turn fatal without medication. The annual maintenance cost with this pricing was around $1,000![4]

Valeant's bid to acquire Allergan was headed off by Actavis, a smaller pharmaceutical company based in Ireland. They purchased Allergan and took the company's name in 2015. The Valeant group later paid $290 million in penalties for insider trading that occurred during the takeover attempt.[5]

In 2019, Allergan was sold to Abbott Laboratories for $63 billion. Abbott immediately spun off AbbVie, a new company for their pharmaceutical business, and it became the new home for Botox and its producer Allergan.[6] AbbVie also marketed a drug that was the world's leading seller at

$19 billion, Humira.[7] The original Abbott would continue to market other health-care products. The arena of finance for big pharma seems to dance to its own tune with an occasional nudge from the government when the "dancers" are out of line.

Formulating, testing, and then obtaining approval for a new drug is a costly proposition. American biopharmaceutical companies are said to spend currently about $1 billion for each new drug that reaches the market.[8] There were fifty approved in 2020. There is no set way that drug development costs are calculated. It remains for the companies themselves to reveal these figures. Sanofi/Regeneron's drug Dupixent, which treats atopic dermatitis and other conditions related to the immune system, was said to have cost $6 billion before approval.[9] This may be a record. In turn, the drug has become a blockbuster in early marketing, selling $5 billion annually with a target of $10 billion.

At the lower end of the scale, minimal cost for drug development has been reported to be $314 million.[10] For an average cost, a more realistic figure may be closer to the aforementioned billion dollars. This is a figure that can be impacted by so many additional costs that it is hard to verify or challenge. Regardless of the amount spent or said to be spent, consistent high standards apply during the drug approval process and are continued throughout the life of the drug as experience with its use is accumulated.

Special consideration applies to so-called orphan drugs that treat rare conditions.[11] To spur approval of these small market but important drugs, certain advantages are offered. These include tax credits for qualified clinical trials, exemption from user fees, and seven years of market exclusivity after approval. In the case of these drugs, though special consideration can be granted for certain administrative issues, standards for safety and quality must be met.

Botulinum toxin type A was approved as an orphan drug with the official US government date of December 29, 1989.[12] The orphan designation carries no stigma. It only recognizes that the drug fulfills an important need, has limited commercial potential, and therefore deserves help. Orphan status was appropriate when Oculinum was first approved for treatment of strabismus and blepharospasm and limited to patients twelve years of age and older. This orphan drug turned into a Cinderella story in a little over a decade as it became a blockbuster, selling well over a billion dollars in a year. With millions of patients worldwide treated, the "orphan" designation remained, but the reason, having a limited market, did not.

How Much Did Alan Scott Spend?

How much did it cost Alan Scott to develop and conduct clinical trials that resulted in FDA approval for Oculinum? The short answer is not much: approximately $4 million.[13] The comparative amount answer is about 1 percent of the lowest developmental cost and .005 percent of the cost of the $6 billion for Dupixent. Scott's expenditure is minuscule when it comes to new-drug development.

Alan Scott broke down the expenses he incurred:

1. Edward Schantz provided the toxin at no cost. At the end of the process, he received a significant royalty once the product was licensed and sold. $750,000.
2. At an early phase, we received a National Institutes of Health grant to support the work at Smith-Kettlewell. This money was used in the sixties and seventies as we examined various toxins over a period of approximately three years. $150,000.
3. Beginning in 1978, the first human received an injection. In 1980, 47 patients were injected with botulinum toxin, and in 1981 an additional 124 were injected. These patients were seen in my private office. Most patients had insurance. This was collected in payment to me for the examination and follow-up, others were seen at no charge because they were volunteering, and their data were valuable. Of course, there was no charge for the drug or the injection procedure. Value not declared.
4. My part-time job at Smith-Kettlewell provided a secretary, laboratory space, and access to core technical help. It is estimated that the worth of this was $80,000 annually. This supported the project from 1980 to 1990. $800,000 in kind.
5. By 1982 it was clear this project would take off and be of clinical value. Because no Big Pharma company would take on botulinum toxin type A as a drug, Oculinum Inc. was established. I took out a $400,000 loan on my house. This was mostly for backup, and only a small amount was used. Not counted as an expense.
6. The major funding for the botulinum toxin clinical trials, between 1982 and 1987, came from donations. Participating doctors were given the opportunity to donate $25 per 100-unit vial for the drug we supplied to them. Donations were received from approximately 21,000 vials through 1986. This raised $525,000. After that it was suggested that donations be increased to $40 per hundred-unit vial. From the next 40,000 vials used, until licensure to Allergan at the end of 1989, we raised $1,600,000. It was clear to us that this was an unusual mechanism for the support of drug development. $2,125,000.
7. At the end of the experimental phase, after licensure, various laboratory personnel who had been working on the hope that more money would be available, were paid in aggregate. $1,000,000.

This was the actual development cost including the time between 1971 and 1990. The ten years of basic research to learn more about the function and behavior of the extraocular muscles and to perfect techniques with electromyography were not factored into the development costs, but they did provide a good start for the program.

The best cash outlay estimate for the cost to develop Botox is roughly $4,025,000.

19

Botox and Beauty

Eighteen minutes to explain a new concept.

D r. Jean Carruthers is an ophthalmologist who learned about botulinum toxin type A from Alan Scott early in her career. Through colossal effort and persistence, she created a virtual empire. Collaborating with her husband, Alastair, she has traveled the world teaching and sharing her experience using botulinum toxin for cosmetics and aesthetics. She spoke at a TEDx talk in her hometown of Vancouver, British Columbia, Canada, on February 13, 2013.

The lights come up in the small auditorium framing the stage; applause from the unseen audience is heard. Entering stage left is the typically attired TED speaker.[1] She is trim and attractive, with short blond hair parted in the middle. She moves to the center of the stage and, with measured steps, wheels slightly to her right to face the audience.

The speaker is dressed in slightly rumpled black trousers and black shoes like a basketball referee wears. Her white blouse is untucked and showing below her waist in front. Over it she wears a dark-blue V-neck sweater. A stand-up, white, starched collar frames a short single strand of large white pearls at her throat. White cuffs of her blouse surround her wrists. A perfectly scripted, casual pose, mostly in black, is achieved—obsidian.

Her face is flawless, without a wrinkle. This speaks volumes, and she has not uttered a word. Those in the audience who bothered to check find it hard to reconcile the speaker with her age—they know she is sixty-five. Her brows are perfectly arched, and her lips are full. Her name is spelled out on the screen behind her for the benefit of the audience. It says, "Dr. Jean Carruthers."

A small black microphone in front of her mouth moves with her head. At the center of the stage, she offers her left hand, acknowledging her audience. Then, with palms up, she silently beckons. *Come with me.* She will tell her story without a formal introduction. The audience knows her name. She begins.

"I'm an ophthalmologist, and my husband, Alastair, is a dermatologist. We both are working in Vancouver. So, I have as a topic today to tell you that we developed, we pioneered, the cosmetic use of botulinum toxin, which most of you know as Botox."

Gesturing to the audience, she asks, "How many of you know Botox? Show your hands. Oh, almost everybody. Probably most of you think it's kind of a yucky sort of vanity drug. Maybe you think about the silver screen starlets on the red carpet or maybe the sort of thing that dismayed people would do, something so frivolous. So, my job today is to teach you the bigger story of this amazing molecule. I will take you from thinking botulism toxin is a terrible poison to its being transformed into a superb new multipurpose drug.

"Now, would you believe me if I told you that this whole story began with sausages and they weren't even good sausages, they were bad sausages? I want you to come back in time with me. I want you to come back to 1822, where in Germany, it is a horrible time in the aftermath of the Napoleonic Wars. There is poverty, there is hunger, and people are still getting together. But most horrifyingly, they're starting to die of an unstoppable paralysis, again and again, and it was terrifying to those people.

"At this time, Justinus Kerner was a German medical officer, and he was so horrified by this—I am too—that he began to study all the outbreaks. After doing this, he concluded it was started by those darn sausages. That was the common factor, and he knew there was something awful in them. But even during all that tragedy, he said, 'I wonder if it would be possible to find out what that was by studying the sausage? What is that little substance in the sausages that is causing all the trouble?' After he got most of the answers he was seeking, he got another idea. 'Maybe we could use that bad thing from the sausage to treat humans who have overactive muscles.' That's a bright idea to come up with in the middle of all that fear and panic.

"Now, move ahead 150 years, going from Germany to San Francisco. In San Francisco is Doctor Alan Scott. He is another ophthalmologist, but he's a genius and he was thinking this: 'I have this great new idea to be able to treat people who have crossed eyes (misaligned eyes) in a new way, instead of doing surgery. What I want to do is to inject something delicately into those eye muscles, changing how they act, so that the muscles will now function to straighten the eyes.'

"And he knew about Justinus Kerner. He knew that this man had even thought of a medical application for this disgusting poison, botulism toxin. So that was one of his choices and he chose three other drugs because he said to me in an email, he thought it was a little weird to just pick Justinus Kerner's molecule.

"Scott did a monkey experiment, injecting eye muscles with tiny doses, billionths of a gram of botulinum, and the other three drugs. But the winner was the botulinum because the monkeys got a predictable change in their eye alignments, and they were perfectly healthy afterward. So being the superb scientist that he is, he's enormously credible, he applied for permission, received it, and began using this medication on humans in a carefully controlled study.

"After that, Dr. Scott moved ahead with his project. It was at that point, in 1982, that I arrived in San Francisco to be his academic fellow. He taught me how to do all the injections and explained so much about anatomy. I was aware though, that as fascinating as it was, I was being introduced to a world that was different from a lot of the people out there. Alan Scott, the genius behind botulinum toxin for the human, had worked out that all that was needed was billionths of a gram to make it safe but still effective. It is a drug, and those out there were still thinking about botulinum as a terrible poison. Not only that, but it was also the most poisonous poison. So there was an air of, shall we say, controversy when I brought the idea back to Canada and applied to Health Canada to join Alan's multicenter study. I would be joining a trial of botulinum to treat misaligned eyes and eye spasms. They granted it to me.

"Now, I slipped in a new condition, and I haven't told you about it. Does anybody know someone who looks like . . ." (*She tilted her head sharply to the left, demonstrating a grimacing face, with forcefully closed eyes.*)

"This distorted face you see, with painful spasms, is what is called *dystonia*. I'm going to call it eye spasms because that's really where we started. So, these people can't live an independent life. To demonstrate, I'm going to share a story with you about Ed, one of my first dystonia patients. His eye spasms had been getting worse and were to the point where he couldn't even get his eyes open at all. He couldn't drive his car. You can't cross the street like this or earn a living with a condition like this. He was led into my office by his wife, his lovely wife. She was desperate too.

"You can imagine Ed's courage in allowing me to inject the shiny new idea, this drug, into his facial muscles to alleviate the spasm. It took tremendous will on his part. So, I treated him, and I got his letter a few days later. It was a thank-you and a picture of him driving his red convertible. How does that feel? That felt amazing to me because his face looked normal in the picture, his eyes were open, and he was happy again, leading an independent life.

"We knew what the treatment, the alternative treatment, for this condition was. It was surgery to pull out the branches of the facial nerve. This can leave a person with an expressionless face and eyelids that don't close, which is quite a bad trade. So, he was thrilled. I was thrilled, and more, I was so enthused. And you know, the thing about these eye spasm patients is a lot of people didn't know what they had. But the eye spasm patients I had treated would go up to these people and say, 'Excuse me, I know what you have, and this is who you should go to see.' There were many patient referrals, and we got very busy.

"The second patient I want to share with you is unusual because she was a severe eye spasm patient returning after what I thought was a successful treatment. She got angry with me, saying, 'You didn't treat me *here*!' and she pointed to vertical frown lines between her eyes. I said to her, 'I'm so sorry, I would have treated you there, but I didn't think that you had any spasm.'

"This episode, and what happened after, pointed out to me that you have to listen to your patients. The patient continued, 'No, I'm not spasming there,' pointing between her brows, 'but every time you treat me, I get this beautiful untroubled expression.'

"Now, I could have ignored that except I'm married to Alastair. Alastair, the dermatologist, had said the treatment for these deep frown lines like those of my unhappy patient are really not good. He had told me he couldn't seem to make anything really work for these patients. With this I said, 'Why don't we do a study with my botulinum and your wrinkle patients?'

"We started. It sounded logical, so we did sort of a study. The first patient we treated was Kathy, who is our wonderful receptionist. Kathy was knowledgeable. She had sat in the office for four years, checking in all my eye spasm and eye alignment patients. She had seen that our patients were always on time, always polite, and always grateful to have their eyes open again. Kathy said sure, so we treated her, and in three days, she got the same result my blepharospasm patient had. Her forehead was smooth, the brow was elevated, and she had a refreshed, open, younger expression. She thought that was great, and after her, we started trying to enroll more people.

"This is where we ran into a problem. People said to us, 'You want to inject what?' We heard, 'Isn't that a poison?'

"There was just too big a gap between what we were offering and what people were able to accept. This prompted us to do the logical thing. We injected me! And if you look now, what do you think? (*She pulls her hair back off her forehead.*) I haven't frowned since 1987.

"We put the study together, and we presented it in 1991 at the American Society for Dermatologic Surgery. We were met with a hailstorm of disbelief, disapproval, and incredulity. We were told, 'You're using that horrible poison on these wrinkle patients.' They said, 'What's wrong with you?'

"But remember, I now had eight years of experience in using this marvelous new drug on patients. I knew it was really restoring their lives to them. So, we decided that if there is this credibility gap, we need to do more research with more publications and more teaching. After doing this, gradually we were invited all around the world to give these talks. We were asked: How do you do it? Why do you do it? Where do you do it? and What are the complications? These are what you expect when you offer something new in medicine. We responded, and gradually all these people started publishing and teaching on their own.

"We got a movement started, and it's growing around the world now. Botulinum treatment has gone from 'you're gonna do what?' or 'that's a crazy idea that will go nowhere' to a procedure that is mainstream. Last year [2012] six million cosmetic injections around the world. It's the number one cosmetic treatment in the world. It is so mainstream now it's a noun, a verb, and an adjective. It's really an amazing change in reputation, but it took twenty-five years of hard work.

"This spring, we were humbled by being given the highest award the American Academy of Dermatology can give for innovation and leadership. It's nice to be recognized while you're still alive.

"Should we go back to the molecule? Maybe yes. It is a molecule that is still giving us messages. The clearest message that we get from this molecule is telling us to look again, and the second message we get is to look deeper. The reason I'm so proud of the cosmetic indication and the cosmetic success of botulinum toxin is because you can't treat six million people in the world without having other doctors in other specialties notice. And there are a number of really interesting new uses. There are now twenty-five government-approved indications in eighty-five countries around the world. That's enormously mainstream.

"Who are these other people who have now moved into the botulinum world? The neurologists are treating spasticity. They are also treating pain syndromes and multiple sclerosis. They also have a particular interest in migraine. How many of you have migraine? I see there's quite a few. That is a miserable condition because you can't think through pain, and you have to take time off in order to recover. Migraine affects about one in eight of the North American population, costing the economy over $50 billion a year in lost income. That's a pretty impressive new use for botulinum.

"What about the dermatologist? They're already using it cosmetically. But how about the excessive sweating that stops people feeling comfortable about shaking hands or attending a meeting because they must wear black or it's just a big pool of sweat? What about the orthopedic surgeons? They're starting to use it, and what about the psychiatrists? The latest twist is that some are starting to use it to treat depression that is said to affect 20 percent of the US population.

"The thing that we did by establishing the cosmetic use was to lay the framework for other specialties to get into this whole idea. People are now thinking, *Okay, I can use it to treat conditions I didn't actually know I could treat before.* I want to thank those early patients and acknowledge them for their bravery and for their trust in letting me inject them. We would not be anywhere near where we are now if it wasn't for their incredible courage and trust.

"Now, what is the other message the botulinum molecule tells us? It's about how to cope with a new idea. New ideas will always be with us. The thing with the botulinum molecule is it was easy to say it's just a poison and write it off. But that wasn't allowed to happen, and it became a brand-new idea. We should really look at new ideas, and we should listen carefully. We should then use our imagination. Let's not forget to do that. We must be prepared to give new ideas a chance. If there is promise, we can't be afraid to put our shoulder to the wheel to do the huge amount of work that is necessary to prove an idea was good. It was a lot of work to prove the worth of botulism for the indication I described today. I was thinking that this botulinum story is a perfect example of this year's TED theme, which is confluence. A terrible poison translates into a superb new drug and a couple of Canadian physicians educate lots and lots of people around the world for the health and well-being of millions.

"I thank you."

Nine years after this TEDx talk, both botulinum toxin and Dr. Jean Carruthers are going strong. We met again in January 2022, this time via Zoom.[3] She was the same vivacious woman and still had that smooth forehead that has not frowned since 1987. The number of people treated worldwide with cosmetic Botox continues to increase, and, as she predicted, the number of therapeutic uses for botulinum toxin has continued to grow.

The drug is firmly established as a multibillion-dollar industry and much of this phenomenal growth can be attributed to the Doctors Carruthers who have carried out clinical research and published and traveled to spread the word in an authentic and convincing way. In the fourth edition of *Procedures in Cosmetic Dermatology*, they write: "Earlier editions talked about botulinum toxin whereas now we are discussing neuromodulators . . . it reflects how we are using the neurotoxins now."[2] This story is an example of the best that can happen in medical discovery.

20

Dermatology Opens the Floodgates

A novel treatment is introduced in an established practice.

In the early years of the development of botulinum toxin, its effect on the skin of the face, where it reduced wrinkles, was noted by Alan Scott and a few others. The effect was obvious, but its significance was not recognized or fully appreciated. This indifference would not last long. By 2002, Botox was approved for cosmetic use in the United States, a year after it had been approved in Canada. Botox, for a variety of cosmetic indications, grew rapidly and resulted in a market representing 50 percent of all Botox sales. How can this drug affect the practice of dermatology? A visit to a busy office to speak with a dermatologist who had expertise in all phases of the specialty proved a good place to start.

It was Friday at 9:00 a.m., in November 2021. Not just any Friday—it was Black Friday, the day after Thanksgiving, when retailers hope to be firmly established with black ink filling the ledgers. It was a rare weekday when this usually bustling medical office was eerily quiet and devoid of staff and patients. Only the lights needed for C. William "Bill" Hanke and me to get around were on. We settled at a table in a conference room to talk.

I first met Dr. Hanke nearly forty years ago, when his dermatology clinic shared a waiting room area with the ophthalmology clinic in the Regenstrief Building at Indiana University Medical Center, where I taught and saw patients. Scarcely ten years out of his residency training in Cleveland, Hanke was a dermatologist who was already becoming a legend for his expertise with a new treatment method for skin cancer called Mohs surgery. This was a game-changing technique: it improved both survival and postoperative appearance in patients treated with surgery for the two most common forms of skin cancer. Now it is state-of-the-art, and Hanke remains a master—but that is not all.

Shifting his practice from the university to the community twenty years ago, Dr. Hanke was the only academician at Indiana University holding professorships in three disciplines: dermatology, pathology, and otolaryngology. While establishing his office in the community, Hanke retained his academic zeal. For a start, he established the only certified outpatient office surgery facility in the state. Then he launched a Mohs surgery fellowship training program. Along the way, he contributed more than four hundred works, including scientific papers, book chapters, and invited papers. He is truly the quintessential man in motion.

Hanke has also been recognized by his peers. He has been president of the International Society for Dermatologic Surgery, the American College of Mohs Surgery, the American Society for Dermatologic Surgery, and the American Academy of Dermatology. He has done it all. Where better to get an informed assessment of the use of Botox and other botulinum toxin drugs than from this dermatologist? I was eager to learn.

According to Hanke, "The use of botulinum toxin—and I include Botox, Dysport, Xeomin, Jeuveau [and there are others]—is strongly rising every year. Botulinum toxin is utilized for cosmetic and therapeutic indications by dermatologists, plastic surgeons, ophthalmologists, otolaryngologists, neurologists, and others.

"Botulinum toxin is on the program of nearly every dermatologic meeting. The physicians who speak are often those whose practices are principally cosmetic dermatology. Botulinum toxin and fillers may represent the majority of some of these practices, whereas it represents only ten to fifteen percent of my practice. I utilize botulinum toxin for treating patients daily for cosmetic facial rejuvenation, axillary hyperhidrosis, temporomandibular joint pain, grinding and clenching of the jaw, and headaches, both migraine and tension. I rarely report on my experience with botulinum toxin at meetings, although I am involved as an investigator on several clinical trials for various cosmetic indications and for axillary hyperhidrosis. Our current Allergan trial targets platysma bands for neck rejuvenation. I was the lead investigator on the US trial for Xeomin produced by Merz, Frankfurt, Germany.

"Patients are nearly always satisfied if botulinum toxin is administered by an experienced, trained physician. Botulinum toxin is also administered by nonphysicians, including nurse practitioners, physician's assistants, and aestheticians, in medical spas and other nonmedical venues. Lesser trained individuals will have more complications. Common complications of botulinum toxin treatment [are due mainly to the site of injection and the amount of toxin injected]. These include upper eyelid droop from inadvertent injections of the levator, upper lid dysfunction due to overtreatment of the orbicularis, and oral dysfunction due to inadvertent injection of a muscle around the mouth.

"Most of my botulinum toxin patients are women, they are of all ages, but some men also have treatment. Botulinum toxin is part of the minimally invasive trilogy, which also includes fillers and lasers. Many patients have all three on a regular basis. One of the positive aspects of minimally invasive treatment has been an accelerated interest in facial anatomy by dermatologists. We understand the location and the function of facial muscles and how to target or avoid them when injecting botulinum toxin. A newer area of interest is facial shaping. For example, the lower face can be narrowed achieving feminization by injecting the masseters with botulinum toxin.

"Botulinum toxin is a multibillion-dollar industry with several companies involved, including AbbVie (branded Allergan), Merz, Galderma, Evolus, and others. Botulinum toxin for facial rejuvenation lasts four to six months. Many patients return for retreatment at four-month intervals. A newly approved botulinum toxin is said to last six months. It has not been marketed to us yet. Patients generally want to look their best, so the future for botulinum toxin is bright with an anticipated continued growth in sales."[1]

Then there is the other side of the coin.

Dr. Hanke added, "I personally have complications from botulinum toxin [but] infrequently. When this occurs, it is possible to lose the patient after the complication resolves. Similarly, I received many new patients after they incur complications from botulinum toxin at the hands of another physician or nonphysician. The companies regularly hold courses and in-office teaching for botulinum toxin techniques for nonphysicians. Some dermatologists, plastic surgeons, and others have nonphysician injectors on site. My practice differentiates itself by [adhering to] physician-administered injectables."

Dr. Hanke and Dr. Jean Carruthers represent two contrasting experiences with a new drug or treatment modality being introduced in medicine. In Dr. Carruthers' case, though fully trained as an ophthalmologist, she was near the beginning of her career when she was introduced to a novel treatment in 1982. At the time, she was an academic fellow in the laboratory and office of Alan Scott, who was carrying out clinical trials for botulinum toxin type A. This toxin was only remotely associated with the primarily cosmetic use that would be developed and promoted by this student, who would later say, "It made wrinkles go away!"

In the case of Dr. Hanke, he was already a professor and renowned expert in the field of Mohs surgery and highly skilled in other areas of the field. He encountered this new treatment near midcareer—not unlike Alastair—and at a time when he had established a secure niche in the field. As a forward-looking physician, he embraced a new and promising technique. He continues to use it for the benefit of the patients he treats. And even more, he serves as a teacher and clinical researcher contributing to the fund of knowledge about this new treatment modality. For this specialist, already practicing as a subspecialist in an exacting surgical field, botulinum toxin is a complement to the range of services he provides to his patients. He proudly explains that botulinum toxin, along with the other facets of facial rejuvenation, is a significant part of the care he offers.

This behavior is common throughout medicine, especially as advances occur and new methods are developed. In the case of botulinum toxin, its acceptance is increasing, but the need for development of new skills for its use is also being recognized. In a survey of dermatology residency training programs, about half responded. Of those, 94 percent said that some cosmetic training using botulinum toxin was offered. However, 38 percent said that this type of training should not be a necessary part of their program. Of those not responding, it is tempting to suspect that most, if not all, did not offer training with botulinum toxin.[2]

The American Society for Dermatologic Surgery offers a one-year fellowship program for training in cosmetic dermatologic care.[3] It does not have board status. This is common with other subspecialties, but membership does have clout. Fellows train with mentors and participate in three hundred cosmetic dermatologic cases and observe one thousand cases all under direct supervision of a fellowship director in at least five of eight categories. In addition, didactic instruction is offered, and fellows are exposed to writing and reviewing clinical manuscripts. Twenty-six fellows were trained in the 2019–2020 calendar year. The Jean and Alistair Carruthers Award is given to the fellow who presents the highest-scoring abstract at the annual meeting.[4]

This type of fellowship training, usually requiring at least an additional year, is available in many medical specialties. This creates a subspecialty culture according to practice but not always certification by an official board. Additional training in a selected area takes place in specialties like ophthalmology, otolaryngology, urology, and many others. The plastic surgeon uses botulinum toxin for a wide range of aesthetic and nonaesthetic indications including wound healing. Today it is common for doctors who have completed residency training covering all aspects of the discipline to select a part of the specialty and secure additional training to become a subspecialist. The generally trained resident is not excluded from the subspecialty area of practice, but it often turns out that this becomes a self-imposed restriction. This is an example where an individual's decision-making is personal and not ruled by arbitrary guidelines and structure.

The groundbreaking efforts of Drs. Jean and Alastair Carruthers, with clinical studies and medical education promoting the use of Botox for cosmetics, opened the floodgates for Botox. The openness of firmly established experts, like Dr. Bill Hanke and others willing to include botulinum toxin treatment in an already established practice, has firmly placed the drug developed from botulinum toxin as a vital tool for the dermatologist willing to acquire the skills to use it. Today, each year, two dozen doctors, after completing a three-year residency training to become a dermatologist, select a one-year fellowship in cosmetic dermatology. Botox and the other neurotoxins, or as some prefer to call them *neuromodulators*, are here to stay.

Some regular uses for Botox (and other botulinum products) by dermatologists include:[5,6]

Asymmetry around the mouth Creating unwanted appearance

Axillary hyperhidrosis Excessive underarm sweating

Blepharospasm Forceful unwanted contraction of eyelids

Crow's feet Lines radiating in the skin from the lateral corner of the eyes

Drooping lid Mild blepharoptosis on one side treated by weakening a closure muscle in that eye

Forehead lines Horizontal lines in the forehead accentuated on looking up

Hemifacial muscle spasm Spasticity of muscles in half of facial muscles or areas adjacent

Glabellar lines Vertical furrows called "frown lines" running perpendicularly between the brows

Golf ball chin Excessive dimpling of the chin

Gummy smile Exaggerated elevation of the upper lip exposing the gum

Masseter muscle enlargement Causing a square face; not feminine

Meige syndrome Forceful contraction of the muscles of jaw and tongue combined with blepharospasm

Migraine Severe headache depending on frequency and duration

Palmar hyperhidrosis Sweaty palms

Platysma hypertrophy Bands standing out in the neck

Salivary (parotid) gland enlargement Creating unwanted square face

Straight low brow Raise brow to create a feminizing arch

The expanded number of conditions that have been considered for treatment with Botox or equivalent may be evidence that anywhere acetylcholine is functioning in the body could be considered for targeted treatment. Two of these include depression and generalized pain.[7]

Many of the indications for botulinum toxin treatment in dermatology are also associated with combined treatment employing, in addition, a filler and laser treatment. Dr. Hanke stressed that dermatologists using botulinum toxin for cosmetic purposes should have a detailed knowledge of the structure of the face. This makes it possible to make small adjustments in the location of injection and the dose of toxin based on experience and the assessment of need while realizing that each patient presents a unique challenge. As with many things in medicine—and in life, for that matter—it helps to have that certain special sense of knowing the right thing to do at the right time. This applies to treatment with botulinum toxin, especially for something that is so much in the eye of the beholder—the patient seeking cosmetic treatment. It is likely that with added experience those who are receiving the treatment will become savvier and those who provide treatment will become more proficient. It is also important to differentiate a complication from an unrealized and possibly unattainable expectation that could have been avoided with realistic pretreatment explanation.

Will there be long-term adverse effects yet to be encountered? That is becoming less likely. It is now more than thirty years since the drug has been approved for medical use, with a growing number of approved indications. And it has been twenty years since it was approved for cosmetic use. Tens of millions have received botulinum toxin treatment, and there have been only a few reports of adverse effects. Most of those effects are related to reaction at the injection site, toxin spread, and flu-like symptoms related to ingredients associated with the toxin—all of which are remedied by time and supportive measures and resolved without lingering effects.

21

Botox and Neurology

A hands-on approach creates effective new ways to treat.

While Alan Scott broadened his own experience with botulinum toxin, he also communicated with other clinicians and clinical researchers. During Scott's drug trials in the 1980s, one of the doctors he welcomed was Joseph Jankovic, professor of neurology and distinguished chair in movement disorders at Baylor College of Medicine. After this visit to Scott's clinic, Jankovic continued to treat an ever-increasing number of different neurologic conditions using Oculinum. He shared this experience in his publications and teaching while gaining preeminence in this area of medicine.

Jankovic's results supported the belief that botulinum toxin is a safe and effective way to treat neurologic disease by controlling overacting muscles. It was a tool with an expanded list of indications. It could do more than treat eye muscles and other spastic muscles around the head and neck. The toxin's ability to block acetylcholine release affected nerve connection and muscle response *anywhere* in the body. For a targeted result, it was only necessary to inject the right dose in the proper place. This made the toxin's effect generic, and it was no surprise to Alan Scott.

In this scenario, developing Botox can be compared to inventing the needle and thread for sewing on a button and then later discovering that this method could be used to connect lots of things—even an entire wardrobe. Scott was not hemmed in by tunnel vision that limited him to the specific objectives of his project, treating strabismus. He adopted a broader outlook. This led him to use botulinum toxin for treatment beyond eye muscles. It started with blepharospasm and other hyperexcitable muscle action mostly around the head. Then straying some, Scott injected the toxin in patients with hip, arm, and leg spasticity in cerebral palsy. He also recognized the toxin's wrinkle-reducing properties, but he said famously, "I just wasn't interested." However, he did make it possible for this avenue to be championed by others.

No field in medicine was more eager to exploit the value of botulinum toxin than neurology. Dr. Scott recounted, "Dr. Joe Jankovic came to Smith-Kettlewell and after that completed the first double-blind placebo-controlled study on patients with blepharospasm." Scott explained that Dr. Jankovic, after this initial work, treated and reported on the treatment of an array of neurologic conditions. At the same time, Dr. Andrew Blitzer, an otolaryngologist from Columbia University in New York, showed that the toxin worked for laryngeal spasm (spasmodic dysphonia). Many more innovators and early adapters in other specialties followed.[1] These renowned specialists would lead, but not be exclusive in, this expanded use of Oculinum during the trials and Botox afterward. New applications were tried in a wide range, from urology to dentistry and beyond and most were effective.

A UNIQUE INDICATION OF INTEREST

Shortly after beginning my participation in the open clinical trial, I was enlisted to coordinate the medical educational experience on a two-week African safari for a group of physicians from various specialties. The tour was focused on sightseeing as well as cross-cultural awareness that included visiting various hospitals and clinics. Attendees would be eligible for additional continuing medical education credits by attending lectures given by me on the bus rides between stops or in a room made available in a facility where we could congregate in the evening. Most attendees were accompanied by their spouse, so one of my challenges was to provide enough varied content to offer something for everybody.

As a pediatric ophthalmologist, my only qualification for this job was that I taught medical students and residents, giving regular lectures on clinical subjects. My own experience in this narrow medical sub-specialty was not a natural fit for a general-medicine audience. I did my best to find topics with some common ground with the group, which included doctors with a wide range of interests. I knew nothing about their spouses.

The history of botulinum toxin and the drug trials underway was a natural for one of the talks. After the lecture, I heard from four physicians representing different areas of medicine. Each said they could think of a use for the toxin to treat conditions encountered in their own practice. They were looking forward to learning more when the drug received FDA approval. Since I had said nothing in the lecture to "sell" anyone on the use of the toxin, I was pleasantly surprised to hear this. I had not expected this level of enthusiasm. I suspect the group would have said more, including the wives, if I had commented on the cosmetic use, but this role of botulinum toxin had not yet become mainstream.

THE NERVOUS SYSTEM

Humans have a nervous system with two major structural components. They are the brain and spinal cord (central) and a series of nerves sending messages to and from the brain (peripheral).

The brain, a structure weighing about three pounds, sits atop the spinal cord and controls all nerve functions in the body, including mentation, pain, voluntary and involuntary movements. It tells us what parts of us, like our feet, are doing when we are not looking (proprioception).

The peripheral nervous system is an array of human "wires" that if placed end to end would stretch to forty-five miles.[2] Impulses scurry about the body, making their way to and from the brain.[3] The peripheral nervous system includes the autonomic and somatic systems.

The autonomic system controls smooth muscle and complex heart muscle, and is working or at the ready always. It regulates a wide variety of body functions without our telling it so. It acts on our behalf when we are asleep, and also when we are awake should our situation call for a specific response. It has two parts, the parasympathetic and the sympathetic. In their actions these systems are diametric opposites. The autonomic system affects a variety of processes including, heart rate, blood pressure, urination, pupil size, digestion, and blood pressure to name a few.

The *parasympathetic/enteric* component slows the heart rate, helps empty the bladder, aids in digestion, causes salivation, and more. It supports the body at rest including digestion.

The *sympathetic* part increases heart rate, slows digestion, dilates the pupils, dilates bronchi for more efficient breathing, causes goose bumps and more. It serves the body in times of stress and danger.

The *somatic* nervous system controls voluntary body movements through action of the skeletal muscles. A person dresses, combs her hair, walks the dog, and smiles or frowns using muscle action mediated by the somatic voluntary system. It is also at work during reflex muscle function. Tap the tendon just below the kneecap with a reflex hammer, and the quadricep muscle receives a somatic nerve impulse to contract and the leg raises.

Acetylcholine is an organic compound that is a neural transmitter functioning as a key element to muscle contraction. As an essential part of the nervous system, it delivers an excitatory nerve impulse in the form of a secretion at the nerve ending. This connector travels to the muscle causing it to contract. You could say acetylcholine is what makes it happen! Without it, healthy nerves and normal muscles fail to connect and produce the intended contraction—paralysis of these muscles occurs. This is what happens in a case of botulism poisoning. The role of acetylcholine has been compared to a plug that connects a perfectly working lamp to a functioning electrical outlet. If that plug, call it acetylcholine, is defective, even with adequate electricity and a perfectly good lamp, there is no light, call it muscle contraction.

Botulinum toxin is a molecule that shuts down the supply of acetylcholine by blocking its production. It first affects the parasympathetic system causing drooping lids, dilated pupils, and difficulty swallowing before moving down from the head to the body to begin affecting somatic muscles. With undiluted Botulinum toxin present in the circulation, an untreated victim is likely to die from respiratory failure in hours to days. Fortunately, with safe food and effective response available today, mortality is around three percent and usually no more than one hundred cases are reported annually. But this same toxin, used in dilutions of billionths of a gram and injected in a specific location, becomes a valuable tool for the management of neurologic disease associated with overacting, spastic muscles.

Technology has enabled the physician to better understand the form and function of the nervous system. This is made possible by devices capable of sophisticated imaging providing accurate recording techniques that depict heretofore inaccessible anatomy and provide information about function in these areas.[4] With these aids it is possible to uncover formerly inaccessible hidden pathology and then deliver targeted treatment. Advances like these are helping neurologists with stroke management and treatment of a variety of other conditions.

Electromyography (EMG) is a basic tool used by the neurologist and others for assessing the status of nerve signal to muscle activity and to locate a muscle not easily palpated from the surface. It can also be a guide for injection in deeper tissue. This procedure was a mainstay for Alan Scott and was a stimulus for his development of Teflon-sheathed needles. However, knowledge of anatomy and observation and experience with botulinum toxin enables accurate injection without EMG in many cases. For the neurologist, botulinum toxin provides a minimally invasive way to treat a variety of nervous system disorders. It does so by temporarily blocking the action of a hyperactive or spastic muscle. It also works well for reasons not well understood as in the case of migraine.

THE EARLY DAYS

In the 1950s, a time when Alan and I were toiling in medical school, the field of neurology as a stand-alone specialty was relatively new. It became established at the department level after World War I at the more forward-looking medical schools and had begun to separate from the specialty of psychiatry, which would also be given department status. Though his first choice for a medical career was cardiac surgery, Scott's fallback was neurosurgery. His thirty-year quest that culminated in FDA approval of Oculinum, followed by the success of Botox, is testimony of Alan Scott's passion for understanding the nervous system.

The neurologist, before the advent of sophisticated imaging, had much in common with the internist. Both dealt with processes occurring throughout the entire body and were not limited to the form or action of a specific part. The internist is concerned with how all systems, including organ function and various interactions, affect any part of the body. The neurologist deals with how stimuli are delivered and received from the brain, muscles, and organs and how these systems respond. Also included is a large variety of sensory information, including pain, as received by the brain. Until recently, tools for investigation by the neurologist were limited, and the treatment consisted mostly of medicines.

The following statement captures the essence of how circumstances have changed for the specialty of neurology: "Until the last couple of decades, when brain studies and other methods of imaging became effective and widespread, neurologists could only observe the consequences of conditions such as Alzheimer's disease . . . and then examine the brain at autopsy. It was like trying to understand how a clock works by watching the movement of the hands [and then] examining the parts after it stops ticking."[5]

Today it is different. A variety of brain and other imaging and function-testing techniques provide the basic scientist as well as the clinician with useful information about the brain and other parts of the nervous system at work. In turn, these images provide new ways to diagnose, interpret, and finally treat many neurologic conditions.

A list of conditions that can be treated with botulinum toxin was compiled by Anandan and Jankovic.[6] This was the result of a literature search supplemented by experience spanning more than thirty years. A common theme for the conditions listed is hyperactivity of a subset of nerves that produce the unwanted symptoms caused by spastic, overactive muscles. In this case, excessive contraction of muscles causing unwanted symptoms is treated with botulinum toxin that blocks acetylcholine, which is essential for muscle contraction. Other conditions also treated by blocking acetylcholine have no muscle involvement at all. This is so for conditions like excessive sweating, where the nerve acts directly on the gland, or migraine, where something similar but yet undescribed is happening. It just works. Relief of symptoms in cases not involving muscles, like axillary hyperhidrosis, can last even longer. This review of indications for the use of Botox compiled by Anandan and Jankovic is based on either evidence-based clinical trials or recent innovative pilot studies.

Blepharospasm This is a sustained involuntary contraction of the muscles around the eye. It is a localized dystonia. This can result in functional blindness simply because the otherwise normally seeing eye is blocked by the closed lids, thereby severely disrupting the life of an individual who is affected. This condition, sometimes called *benign essential blepharospasm*, has no known cause and was one of the first of the expanded uses of botulinum toxin.

Cervical Dystonia the commonest form of dystonia, is a "pain in the neck." It is characterized by involuntary contractions of the neck muscles, leading to sustained abnormal head and neck position along with pain.

Drooling (Sialorrhea) overproduction of saliva by the salivary glands causing leaking from the mouth.

Dystonia This is defined as a movement disorder characterized by sustained or intermittent muscle contraction. It is like spasticity, which is related to hyperexcitability. A combination is called *spastic dystonia*, which is an inability to relax resulting in prolonged contraction.

Flexion of Trunk (Camptocormia) abnormal posture and threat to balance caused by forward bending of the upper body. It can be an isolated finding but is frequently associated with other diseases, such as Parkinson's. This posture increases during walking and goes away when supine (lying on the back).

Hemifacial spasm This is a tonic contraction on one side of the face. It occurs in the area served by the facial nerve and can be caused by pressure on that nerve. The result is an irregular contraction of the muscles on just one side of the face. This is not painful, but it is disturbing to the person affected.

Laryngeal Dystonia a sustained contraction of the vocal muscles leading to either closure or separation of the vocal cords, both resulting in abnormal speech. This can be a strained voice when the cords are held closed and a breathy voice when they are held open.

Limb Dystonia This dystonia in the upper limb is commonly seen as writer's cramp, or it can be task-specific, such as would occur in musician's dystonia that hinders use of a finger to reach a piano key or manipulate the fine workings of an instrument, such as an oboe or clarinet. It can also occur in the foot in the case of a runner.

Lingual Dystonia a rare type of dystonia affecting only the tongue. It is usually associated with a debilitating condition and brought on by eating and noted in patients with neurodegenerative disorders.

Migraine headache attack of four to seventy-two hours; typically unilateral in location, pulsating in quality, moderate to severe in intensity, aggravated by physical activity, and associated with nausea and light and sound sensitivity (photophobia and phonophobia).[7]

Myoclonus involuntary, jerk-like contraction of the muscle. It can be either positive with the muscle acting excessively or negative with a brief lapse of muscle contraction. This can occur in almost any muscle.

Oromandibular Dystonia a focal dystonia that affects the face, mouth, and jaw. This can be expressed by jaw opening or closing or by related bizarre tonic behavior mostly of the tongue.

Parkinson's Disease a neurogenerative disease with a variety of symptoms, including hand tremors, jaw tremors, axial dystonia, freezing gait, drooling, and disrupted voluntary movements.

Restless Leg Syndrome chronic or intermittent neurologic condition characterized by the urge to move lower limbs due to an uncomfortable sensation in the legs.

Tic recurrent, jerk-like, or transitory sustained involuntary movements.

Tremors an involuntary, rhythmic, oscillatory movement of a body part. It is the most common movement disorder.

MIGRAINE

"The prevalence and burden of self-reported migraine and severe headache in the US adult population is high, affecting roughly one out of every six Americans and one in five women."[8] Eleven million, about 3 percent of the population, are moderately to severely disabled by their attacks. This results in significant "lost labor" costs, substantial health care expenses, and a pervasive negative impact on overall quality of life in sufferers. A breakthrough indication for the use of Botox was a boon for those who suffer from migraine or related severe headaches. It is available for those who need it, but a patient does not "drop in" for Botox treatment of migraine. Instead, a thorough evaluation and trial of other treatment is required for this condition to be eligible for coverage by insurance.

Once a migraine patient qualifies for coverage and receives treatment with botulinum toxin, the occurrence of headaches can be reduced by 50 percent and in some cases 70 percent, meaning treatment provides a significant benefit in terms of quality of life which is considerably improved.[9] Treatment intervals vary according to response. They are usually every twelve weeks or approximately four times a year. This treatment is exacting and expensive.

Botox treatment of migraine, according to recommended usage, entails thirty-one injection sites receiving five units each. This is a total of 155 units. Current rules state that any unused toxin be destroyed.

The dots in the figure depict the suggested sites for injection of botulinum toxin to treat migraine headaches. This treatment scheme is modified by some users who use smaller doses in selected, but not all, recommended areas and with satisfactory results.

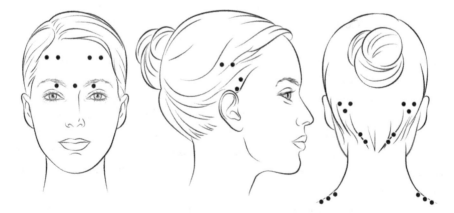

Suggested sites for injection of five units of Botox for the treatment of migraine. Some treaters report success using fewer sites and a slightly different pattern of injection.

Dr. Kristi George has been in private practice as a neurologist for twenty-five years. In keeping with the medical specialty she chose, she has a bachelor's degree in electrical engineering! Dr. George graduated from the Indiana University School of Medicine and completed an internship and neurology residency at the Indiana University Hospitals and clinics. After that she completed a neuromuscular fellowship with Dr. John Kincaid and studied the use of Botox with Doctor Allison Brashear in 1995 and 1996.[10]

Dr. George said, "My first experience with Botox was during training. Not all residents used it then. There were no set rules, and those not interested just didn't use Botox. Not everyone was interested in using it, but I was."[11]

"Since training with botulinum toxin wasn't part of my program and I was interested, I went about learning in the best way I could find. That turned out to be seeking out the staff member who did the most with Botox. That was Doctor Brashear, and I learned from her. She was the lead person with Botox at IU at that time and had published a work on upper limb spasticity. I knew that this training with Botox in neurology was optional, but I did it anyway.

"Botox treatment is one of the things we can really do ourselves for our patients. Traditionally in neurology, we are limited to diagnosis after physical examination and review of laboratory and imaging studies, and then we begin treatment with medicine. There have been a lot of things we can't do. Botox is something that works incredibly well for what we use it for. It provides something I can do for my patients that is hands-on, and that is something which I like. Since we have very few procedures in our practice, having Botox offers us the opportunity to treat the patient physically in the office. That is a good thing.

"I consider using Botox *interventional*. I treat patients who have Blepharospasm, hemi-facial spasm, upper and lower limb spasticity, organic writer's cramp, and of course migraine, which is about half of what we do for treatment now. I also treat muscle spasm, but it's tough to get insurance to cover this treatment. When it could work well, we inject some for pain, but insurance is extremely iffy."

"In the beginning, I used Botox treatment only on a regular 'Botox day,' but now I use it for a handful of patients every day. One problem with Botox is that you cannot share vials between patients. In our cases, if the entire vial is not used for a patient, we throw out the rest in the waste. When it comes to cosmetic use, occasionally a patient will ask if some of the Botox can be used for an 'extra' use treating a wrinkle. That would be a violation of established rules and could result in the entire treatment being disallowed for coverage, so I say no.

"Something that is annoying that the insurance companies do that has no answer is this: for treatment of migraine, some insurance coverage will pay for 155 units but will not pay for anything that goes over this. If you were to give more than 155 units, they would not simply refuse to pay for the additional Botox used; they would pay nothing! Yes, hard to believe but they would pay nothing. At the same time, after you've used your 155 units, you would have to throw the rest away. This just doesn't make sense!"

Dr. George identified the areas of the face, head, and neck where injections were applied in the usual patient. These included around the eyes and forehead, the corrugator, the procerus, frontalis, on the side of the head temporalis, on the back of the head occipital area, the neck or cervical area, and top of the shoulders or trapezius area. Since the potentially lethal dose of Botox in the human is 3,000 units, the 155-unit injection for migraine is still an extremely safe dose.

"In the beginning, there was some concern that the protein binder included with the toxin would cause the production of antibodies. This would mean that further treatments would not be effective, especially when larger doses like those for migraine were given. I don't think this is happening, although some patients don't get as much effect after a while. To be certain no immunity is developing, I inject a place on the forehead. If the response is good, I am confident that no immunity has developed.

"Sometimes patients make an appointment, and it turns out they just want Botox, or they may be referred by another neurologist or by a family physician. Other people who make an appointment [for Botox] may have just heard about it. When it comes to Botox and migraine, which is the most frequent patient indication [in my practice], it is not possible to simply see the patient and start the treatment right away. It is necessary to go through a specified program and protocol before the insurance coverage will pay for Botox."

When asked her thoughts on the future for botulinum toxin, Dr. George's response was, "I don't know. . . . Maybe it would be a new nonorganic, chemical agent, and maybe it would be something that lasts longer.

I can't come up with any new uses offhand, but I am satisfied it works well for the things we are using it for now."

Dr. George and I agreed that the effects of Botox wearing off were not all bad. For example, when a complication occurs, as when an unintended muscle weakness results from a spread of the toxin or a slightly misplaced injection produces a drooping lid or a crooked smile, the effect wearing off is a relief for all. Dr. George concluded, "I am very happy with the results of Botox for everything that I use it for in treating my patients. Getting insurance to pay for pain treatment is very iffy and uncertain. My guess is that about ten percent of neurologists use Botox. A lot of them quit using it because of problems with insurance. The doctors who quit are likely those who lost money because the insurance does not pay consistently."

22

The Legacy

Alan B. Scott: the man who made Botox.

In the fall of 2021, Alan B. Scott was nearing his ninetieth birthday. More than thirty years before, he had established his record of accomplishment and earned respect from the world of science by finding a way to transform the deadliest toxin known into a drug suitable for use in humans. Scott summed up this path to success as follows: "I was pretty good in the clinic and around the lab okay, but I was a lousy businessman." This may have a ring of truth to it, but it fails to account for another of Scott's traits. This was his dogged persistence over a thirty-year span of single-minded effort that it took to fulfill the two-century-old prophecy of Justinus Kerner, who said that the death-dealing fatty poison in blood sausage could have use as a drug in a human.

Alan Scott, who worked without letup, took the final step by transforming a purified toxin used in the laboratory into a versatile drug that helps millions worldwide. It all began with his initial challenge:

Find a way to treat strabismus or misalignment of the eyes by selectively weakening an extraocular muscle with an injection instead of traditional incisional surgery currently employed.

Scott's Path

1961 Began a decade of study to calibrate and describe the action of eye muscles in normal and strabismic humans.

1972 Tested several agents, all of which proved unsatisfactory, for selective muscle weakening. Learned about botulinum toxin, consulted with other researchers about its use in the lab, and finds a source for the toxin.

155

1972–77 Diluted and freeze-dried botulinum toxin, established the mouse unit (LD_{50}) at .73 nanograms, determined the LD_{50} in a 70 kg human would be a safe 3,000 units, changed the stabilizing agent of the toxin to human albumin, and created a toxoid for vaccination to protect researchers.

1973 Reported on injection of botulinum toxin in a primate (monkey) that successfully altered alignment for months using a dose that was a mere fraction of the human LD_{50}, confirming the toxin was safe while observing no side effects. Disclosure eliminated patentability of the drug.

1977 Obtained an Investigational New Drug authorization from the Food and Drug Administration (FDA) to begin human trials.

1978 Became the first person to inject a human with botulinum toxin type A, the world's most lethal toxin.

1980 Reported on first injection of botulinum toxin in a human.

1981 Reported on first large series of human extraocular muscle injections, expanded FDA-authorized drug trials to phases 2 and 3.

1981 Learned that the toxin smoothed wrinkles, reversed blepharospasm, stopped facial spasm, and treated cervical dystonia and limb spasticity in cerebral palsy.

1982–89 Recruited and trained participants in an open trial with ophthalmologists and other specialties while encouraging wider application of the drug.

1982 Encouraged a trainee who subsequently promoted and secured approval of the toxin for use in cosmetics.

1982–83 Established Oculinum Inc. (and named the drug Oculinum) to comply with FDA regulations that biological substances have a legitimate manufacturer.

1983–88 Tried unsuccessfully to sell Oculinum to a pharmaceutical company.

1987 Smith-Kettlewell and California Pacific Medical Center no longer support distribution of botulinum toxin for human use because of concerns with liability. FDA stops Scott's distribution of the toxin.

1988–89 Completed Phase 3 of clinical trials and prepared data for the FDA's new drug application.

1989 Received FDA approval on December 29, 1989.

1990 Licensed Oculinum to Allergan.

1991 Sold Oculinum to Allergan for $9 million. The drug's name was subsequently changed to Botox. Scott had no further contact with Allergan after the sale.

1994 Organized Strabismus Research Foundation (SRF) and publishes results of enhanced Botox effect by adding bupivacaine to weak muscle.

2014 Established Strabismus Research Foundation (SRF) as a not-for-profit corporation and continued project to inject bupivacaine into a paretic muscle and Botox into a normal muscle to enhance effectiveness. Confirmed the effectiveness of this combination.

Through 2021 Remained active as a strabismologist, consultant, and teacher and cooperated in preparation for this book until his death in December 2021.

When Alan Scott found a solution, he avoided grandiose claims. When he reported success, he neither overpromised nor underdelivered. While seeking a new way to treat strabismus without the need for incisional surgery, he set modest and realistic goals and succeeded in the specific areas addressed.

When new uses for botulinum toxin type A were found, mostly defined by how it was employed in a specific specialty, Scott encouraged those involved to pursue their efforts. He was an ophthalmologist and continued to deal with the challenges that were of interest to him, and he dealt with the patients he was called on to treat. That was enough for him. Other reasons for Alan's seeming monomania could be his need to fully understand and maintain control while taking responsibility for what he was doing. Perfectionism could have been his guide. Another explanation for his focus is that so much was coming at him from so many directions, he wanted to organize or compartmentalize the work to give himself a better chance to do the right thing. But this is nothing more than conjecture on my part.

Openness, generosity, sharing, and a sense of accomplishment were foremost with Alan Scott and a perfect example of how Walter Isaacson characterizes most researchers in his book *The Code Breaker*: "All the scientists I write about in this book say that their main motivation is not money, or even glory, but the chance to unlock the mysteries of nature and use these discoveries to make the world a better place . . . reminding scientists of the nobility of their mission."[1]

Jackie Lehmer, Alan Scott's wife, said to me, "It is too bad so many people are unaware that this [Botox] treatment is available because of Alan. They think their own doctor did it."[2]

And Alan Scott would likely have shrugged and said, "So what?"

However, I do agree with her and others who feel that the public knows too little of what Alan Scott accomplished. Thousands of articles written about botulinum toxin mention Alan's role briefly, but the words become perfunctory, making it seem like he happened to be around when Botox emerged.

In the history of the development of Botox, there may be two categories of scientific accomplishment that deserve recognition. One is the purely scientific part advanced by people who dealt with the bacteria and its toxin. These include, in my opinion, Émile Pierre-Marie van Ermengem, Carl Lamanna, Arthur Guyton, Edward Schantz, Karl Meyer, Hermann Sommer, Arnold Burgen, Vernon Brooks, and Daniel Drachman. These researchers worked in their labs in Europe, Canada, and the United States to unlock the mysteries of the toxin. The other class of accomplishment happened on the clinical stage, where botulinum was given a life and a voice. The first voice appeared with Justinus Kerner, and a second voice a century and a half later, with Alan Scott.

The botulinum toxin story has ample room for credit to be shared by those who are acknowledged here, while others who have contributed remain unsung. The breakthrough clinical accomplishments belong to Justinus Kerner and Alan Scott. The single sustaining force was in one man who assembled the parts to create a coherent whole that made possible a new drug to arise from the toxin produced by Ed Schantz. Building on a fund of knowledge assembled by those who studied botulinum toxin for a century and a half, Alan Scott accepted the challenge and took the next giant step when he gave the world a drug that was his own creation.

Alan Scott is a man who deserves to stand at the head of the heroes of the botulinum toxin story. He ran the anchor lap of this race. We remember Neil Armstrong as the first man to walk on the moon, though his efforts were made possible by thousands in the background. The same applies to Alan Scott. He took that fateful, critical step that turned a deadly toxin into a drug to benefit humankind now and in the years to come. When he injected botulinum toxin type A into a human extraocular muscle, this man virtually walked on the moon.

Whatever happens in the future with botulinum toxin, even to there being a synthetic version, the breakthrough resulting in its use in a human remains the crowning achievement of a clinical ophthalmologist working part time as a researcher. He pursued a full-time quest with unwavering effort and saw the job to completion.

Alan Scott made it happen.

Alan Scott's life in three equal parts

1932–1961
Getting started

1962–1991
Taming the world's deadliest toxin and creating Botox

1992–2021
Perfecting who he was and consolidating his accomplishment

RIP

Epilogue

After Alan Scott's death, Botox continues as the juggernaut of the botulinum toxin market with only growth prospects in the foreseeable future. There are other brands: some with innovations like a longer duration, more convenient packaging, and modifications that hold promise but are not yet perfected. After thirty years, adverse results from the drug have been limited, even minuscule. Proper dosing, appropriate indications, and competent injections seem to be the limiting factors, and these seem well in hand. Alan Scott can certainly be fully credited with taming the beast. His long-term prediction that an inorganic form *could* be a possibility is something for the uncharted future. For now, the toxin continues to prosper with the upside that there is a virtually limitless potential for discretionary demand and the drug's effect is transitory. You like the result, and you do it again.

Alan Scott died a half year short of his ninetieth birthday and nearly a week before Christmas. A void was established with many, and that included his widow Jackie Lehmer, who reminisced.

After the sale of Oculinum to Allergan, Alan maintained his interest in all aspects of strabismus—and life, for that matter. In doing so, he sought novel approaches or developed improvements in something that had been done before. He also accepted many invitations to be a speaker at meetings around the world. If any regrets lingered about turning his back on a drug that was beginning to sell in the hundreds of millions and even billions of dollars, it did not show. Why? Because it wasn't there. Jackie Lehmer, who was with Alan for the last twelve years of his life, had never heard a word or suspected a murmur of regret from Alan that he was not awash with the millions that were his due if he had sought them. He didn't care. He had no regrets.

Ever the teacher (or call it problem-solver), Alan was a regular contributor to the pediatric ophthalmology listserv that gave doctors worldwide the opportunity to share challenging patients with colleagues, and even gain the attention of experts. When this happened, Alan was there, offering sage advice based on his wealth of experience.

He had lost his companion Ruth of fifty years, but it turned out because of a friendship developed by Ruth, he found a new companion to be his wife—a friend whom Ruth had been close to for years. This began when Ruth and Jackie were docents at the Academy of Science Museum in San Francisco. Over a period of twelve years, Alan and Jackie each retained the thread of a happy prior life while creating a union that enriched both until Alan's passing. Describing their last Thanksgiving together, Alan proudly announced, "We're twenty-two for dinner and we are feeding them two turkeys and all the rest." These were the words of a happy man. "Alan especially loved Thanksgiving," said Jackie.

In a phone conversation in the summer of 2022, a half year after Alan's death, his widow asked me how the book was coming along. This led to a discussion of how Alan's level of curiosity never waned. She told me this story:

"Alan was working on a project with my grandson who is a planetary astronomer working with NASA. I don't know much about it, but it was about a Hess-Lancaster something." I knew she was talking about a device to chart strabismus angle and that Alan was still working on new ideas. Jackie Lehmer offered to have her grandson call me to explain more about the project, and he did.

Owen Lehmer described what he had been working on with Alan and sent a link to the digital Hess-Lancaster screen that was still in development. On my computer screen, I saw the partially finished program that was a clever, simple, and useful scheme for obtaining an objective measure of a patient's eye alignment. Owen later forwarded six email threads from Alan between October 2020 and June 2021. The partially finished project was sidetracked, but it remains as evidence that Alan Scott was still in the game and never quit.

Appendices

Justinus Kerner

Justinus Andreas Christian Kerner was a polymath who lived a long life in a period of progress. Born in 1786 and dying in his seventy-sixth year in 1862, his life spanned the time from the formation of the United States to the Civil War.[1]

He was born in Ludwigsburg in the South German state of Baden-Württemberg, attending local schools until he apprenticed in a cloth factory. With help from outside the family, he was able to enter the University of Tübingen. There he studied medicine but also pursued literary interests among the scholars there. After graduation he travelled, before settling as a district medical officer in Bad Wildbad. There he began his extraordinary work with botulism poisoning in the state of Wurttemberg. Through his efforts he discovered botulism poisoning was caused by a toxin. Further study of the toxin led him to the prescient statement that it could find a use in medicine. If that had been the end of the contributions of Justinus Kerner, his life would have been one of great consequence. As it turned out, this was only the beginning, or an interlude, in his eventful life.

Shortly after his discoveries with botulism poisoning, Kerner published *Travel Shadows*, a book that was a mixture of poetry and prose, featuring romance, seriousness, and humor. Before beginning his practice of medicine, Kerner had authored a book about his boyhood. Later Kerner studied the works of somnambulists and clairvoyants, which led to his interest in the inner life and hypnotism.

A multifaceted man, Kerner was engrossed in the behavior of not only the natural world but of the supernatural.[2] He was interested in exorcism as a scientific study of disease. These interests were not labeled eccentric at the time; rather, they were commonplace in both Europe and the United States.

Residing in Weinsberg during his second posting as a district medical officer, Kerner continued his seminal work with botulism poisoning and maintained his medical practice. In a parallel way of life, he pursued other interests, remaining in Weinsberg for the rest of his life with family, friends, and patients. He resided in comfortable surroundings with assistance from the help of well-placed friends within the aristocracy who were patrons. Kerner generously opened his home to many who made the pilgrimage to this site.

An enduring accomplishment of Kerner's genius might have been with the practice he devised and called *klecksographs*. These are figures created by inkblots duplicated symmetrically on folded paper. He discovered this as a byplay of unintended drops of ink that occurred while he wrote. When he folded the paper, he noted the interesting figures. They inspired poetry. When the mood struck, he would enhance these figures with small additions that gave more character to the image that was forming in his mind. (See page 81.)

The Rorschach test, used by psychologists today was developed by Hermann Rorschach in 1921. Based on klecksographs as created by Kerner, the Rorschach test is still in use today.

A Poem by Justinus Kerner[3]
The Saw

by Justinus Kerner
Translated and published by
William Cullen Bryant, in the public domain

In yonder mill I rested,
And sat me down to look
Upon the wheel's quick glimmer.
And on the flowing brook.
As in a dream, before me,
The saw, with restless play,
Was cleaving through a fir-tree
Its long and steady way.
The tree through all its fibers
With living motion stirred,
And, in a dirge-like murmur,
These solemn words I heard—
Oh, thou, who wanders hither,
A timely guest thou art!
For thee this cruel engine
Is passing through my heart.
When soon, in earth's still bosom,
Thy hours of rest begin,
This wood shall form the chamber.
Whose walls shall close thee in.
Four planks—I saw and shuddered—
Dropped in that busy mill;
Then, as I tried to answer,
At once the wheel was still

APPENDIX 2

Dr. Karl Meyer

Dr. Karl Meyer was a world-renowned epidemiologist and virologist who played an important role in the story of botulism poisoning. One part of this work led to the discovery of equine encephalitis. In 1930, horses were dying in California's San Joaquin Valley in startling numbers. Up to 10 percent of herds were perishing from a neurologic disease, with numbers totaling in the thousands. The cause was thought to be botulism poisoning.

As the botulism expert from the University of California, Dr. Meyer was sought out for help. He responded by leading a team that observed the afflicted horses. To the disappointment of those requesting his help, Meyer challenged, "If not botulism, what?" Meyer suspected it was some other type of encephalitis. To confirm this, he needed a specimen of a recently ill animal to obtain brain tissue and conduct studies.[1]

At a meeting of the American Association of Immunologists Meyer told this story:

"I told my team to scour the herds searching for an animal recently ill but still alive. I got a call one day in the afternoon, telling me that such an animal has been located in Merced. I was in San Francisco, but said I would be there in four hours. When I arrived at the farm after navigating hours of county roads, I was confronted by a farmer who said he would shoot anybody who got near his horse. This spurred an alternative plan for me. I spoke with the man's wife telling her the horse would be dead within hours and would be worth nothing. I offered the woman twenty dollars for the horse. Then to approach the horse, I told the woman to wait till her husband was asleep; then, she should raise the window shade to let me know that the coast was clear.

That evening, with my small group stationed at the edge of the property I saw the shade go up. By 9:30 it was dark. I scaled a fence, went to the horse barn, and euthanized the dying animal with strychnine. I removed the horse's head and, with the help of my men, transported it several miles to an arranged location: an abandoned chicken coop. There, I carried out the necessary brain dissection, recovering tissue and solutions to begin our studies.

By 5:30 in the morning, we were back in San Francisco in the laboratory. We used the specimens to inoculate an array of laboratory animals to serve as reservoirs for what I suspected was the offending substance. I was able to isolate and identify what would be called the Western equine encephalomyelitis virus. This was the first time this entity had been discovered, and it answered important questions.

A significant result was the vaccination against botulism that was used widely at great cost could now be stopped since it was no longer necessary."

This is an extreme example of a scientist taking matters in his own hand, and acting in a way that would be considered unethical, highly questionable, and even criminal today. In this case, which I suspect is not isolated, good resulted from an act that some would object to.

Western equine encephalomyelitis also affects humans. It occurs largely west of the Mississippi River and is spread by the bite of a mosquito. In the mild form, it produces flu-like symptoms. Fatality is 3 percent. A more virulent disease, eastern equine encephalitis is found east of the Mississippi.

APPENDIX 3

Dr. Arthur Guyton

Dr. Arthur Guyton was born in 1919 in Oxford, Mississippi. He graduated from Harvard Medical School in 1943 after marrying Ruth in his senior year.[1] His plan was to become a surgeon. This was interrupted by a call to active duty in the US Navy. He was stationed first at the National Naval Medical Center in Bethesda, Maryland, then was reassigned to Frederick, Maryland, where he joined a group of young scientists at a new facility called Camp Detrick. These young men would play a significant role supporting the war effort during World War II.

Their job included learning more about botulinum toxin as a threat for biological warfare and coming up with an effective vaccine against its possible use. They accomplished this and more. At twenty-five, Arthur Guyton designed and built laboratory equipment, making it possible for him to study the regulation of skeletal muscle movement within motor neuron terminals. Doing this he also explained the details of neurotransmitter release at the molecular level. This laid the groundwork for the eventual development of medical botulinum toxin type A, now called Botox, based on the work of Alan Scott.[2]

By 1947 and discharged from the navy, Guyton developed polio, with a sustained paralysis that limited him to difficult walking with braces and canes, and a motorized wheelchair of his design for efficient locomotion. This did not stop him; he did not seem to possess a neutral gear. However, it called for a change in career plans, from surgery to physiology and a life of research and teaching.

Arthur and Ruth Guyton returned to Mississippi in 1947 with two babies in tow. They would be the first of ten, including two girls and eight boys. Arthur started teaching in Oxford before the family moved to Jackson when the medical school earned accreditation for a four-year program. Arthur was Chairman of the Department of Physiology, where he remained throughout his distinguished career. In his research, Guyton made breakthrough discoveries about cardiac output, intercellular pressure, fluid retention, and cardiac failure. Among his other signal achievements was an explanation of the role of the kidneys in the fluid control of hypertension.

Stepping out of the laboratory and into the classroom, Guyton wrote his *Textbook of Medical Physiology* in 1956, and it is now in its fourteenth edition. It is the most widely used medical text in the world, and is arguably one of the most successful medical textbooks of all time. But the superlatives do not end there. All ten children of Arthur and Ruth Guyton are medical doctors! Their oldest son, David, is a renowned pediatric ophthalmologist who follows in his father's footsteps as a brilliant inventor. The other nine Doctors Guyton have also carved out distinguished careers.

APPENDIX 4

I Didn't Make the Team

By the early 1990s, we were using Oculinum under its new name Botox and purchasing it from its new owner, Allergan. This was a well-known and trusted company that supplied many of the medicines and other products we used on a daily basis for patient care. The otherwise seamless transition from Alan Scott to the new company was complicated for me by an aversion to the new name. It was something I couldn't explain, but the feeling was real.

As was the practice at the time, we would be visited by an Allergan representative. The initial contact was arranged by one of our staff. Today's encounter would be with a new rep—a woman who was pleasant but made it clear she was all business. As it turned out, she was not there to extol the virtues of one of their products. She had something else on her mind.

After introductions, she said she was here to talk about Botox. I indicated that would be fine with me. This was taking place while our Oculinum—oops, Botox—clinic was in progress. She asked me what kind of patients we were treating, how often they returned, what results we were achieving, and if we were having any problems. I told her most of our patients were seniors suffering from some form of dystonia. Results of treatment with Botox were outstanding; the patients were happy and had experienced no untoward effects. We treated strabismus patients who would benefit from the toxin, but the numbers were small. In all, we were delighted with the drug and happy to have it.

Pleased with what she heard, she proceeded by telling me the real reason for this visit. Allergan was in the process of preparing a new culture of Botox.* The company was nearing the end of the culture they had purchased from Dr. Scott. Moreover, it was time they had their own homegrown supply. As part of this resupply process, Allergan was assembling an oversight panel of physicians and scientists, and the rep was inviting me to be part of that team. My job would be simply to be available to answer any questions the developers might have and to represent the company that was bent on doing the right thing. Finding no reason to decline, I immediately accepted.

Following this, she asked about our charging practices and the financial impact on our practice. When I told her, she developed a frown. I continued saying most of our patients were on Medicare, which did not pay for the treatment. So, we continued a billing policy—more like non-billing—that we employed during the trials. We broke even, more or less, but that was all.

This was not what she wanted to hear. Her response was to tell me that some of her doctors in Florida were charging a thousand dollars for some treatments. She might have said more, but it was while she was turning and walking away from the aborted meeting. With this act, I assumed that whatever I had agreed to was now null and void. To this day that represents my only contact with the company beyond an occasional visit from a rep.

---

*Allergan received FDA approval for a new culture to produce Botox in 1997.

Glossary

A

Abbott Laboratories A multinational medical device and health-care company with headquarters in Abbott Park, Illinois, United States.

AbbVie An American publicly traded biopharmaceutical company founded in 2013. It originated as a spinoff of Abbott Laboratories.

acetylcholine A molecule that is present throughout the body with far-reaching effect, acting as a neurotransmitter.

Actavis Global pharmaceutical company focused on acquiring, developing, manufacturing, and marketing branded pharmaceuticals, generic and over-the-counter medicines, and biologic products.

Allergan An American Irish-domiciled pharmaceutical company that acquires, develops, manufactures, and markets brand-name drugs and medical devices in the areas of medical aesthetics, eye care, central nervous system, and gastroenterology. The company is the maker of Botox for parent company AbbVie Inc.

anaerobic Relating to, involving, or requiring an absence of free oxygen.

antigen A toxin or other foreign substance that induces an immune response in the body, especially the production of antibodies.

antitoxin An antibody that counteracts a toxin.

assay Determination of the pharmacological potency of a drug.

autonomic Involuntary or unconscious; relating to the autonomic nervous system.

B

bacteria Mostly free-living organisms and measuring millionth of a meter.

bacterium Singular of *bacteria*.

biologic Of or relating to biology or to life and living processes.

biological equivalence Biological response as a measure of dose.

blitzkrieg "Lightning war" launched by Hitler in World War II.

blockbuster A drug that has $1 billion or more in annual sales.

blood sausage Links stuffed with blood and a variety of other foods like meat, grain, and fat and cooked in boiling water.

botulism poisoning Acute poisoning caused by botulinum toxin, characterized by muscle weakness and paralysis.

buzz bomb Jet-propelled, pilotless missile Germans used against England in World War II.

C

camptocormia A forward leaning of the upper part of the body when walking or standing.

canning A method of food preservation in which food is processed (usually heated to 240 degrees Fahrenheit) and sealed in an airtight container.

catch-22 A difficult dilemma from mutually conflicting dependent conditions introduced in the book of that title by Joseph Heller.

Celsius A scale of temperature with water freezing at 0° and boiling at 100°.

Centers for Disease Control and Prevention (CDC) National public health agency of the United States.

chain reaction A chemical reaction or other process that promotes or spreads the reaction, sometimes dramatically. The basis for the atomic bomb.

Churchill, Winston Prime minister of Great Britain during World War II.

civil suit A legal action between individuals usually associated with compensation.

Clostridium botulinum A bacterium that produces botulinum toxin.

cohiba cigar A Cuban cigar, favorite of Fidel Castro.

Cold War A state of political hostility that existed between the Soviet bloc countries and the US-led Western powers from 1945 to 1990.

concomitant Same in two places, such as, "The angle of deviation is concomitant in each eye."

conjunctiva A mucous membrane covering the front part of the eye around the cornea and the underside of the eyelids.

consent A key term in medicine meaning a subject understands and agrees to an action or undertaking.

cornea The round clear center "window" at the front of the eye.

corrugator A muscle that draws the eyebrows together and wrinkles the brow in frowning.

D

depth perception The ability to perceive the relative distance of objects in one's visual field and the ability to see objects in three dimensions.

dystonia Muscular spasm.

E

electromyography Recording of electrical activity when nerves excite muscle contraction.

endotoxin Moderately toxic and is liberated when the bacterium dies.

Escherichia coli A bacterium commonly associated with undercooked meat, causing diarrhea and cramps.

exotoxin Highly toxic protein secreted or released by pathogenic bacteria.

exotropia Outward deviation of one or both eyes; sometimes called "walleyed."

F

Fahrenheit A scale of temperature on which water freezes at 32 degrees and boils at 212 degrees.

forceps A delicate grasping device.

Fresnel prism A thin lightweight prism comprised of multiple small prisms that together have the same power as a single large prism of the same angle.

frontalis Forehead muscle that raises the eyebrows.

G

gram positive A staining designation for identifying bacteria.

gravity sled An informal device to create and measure the centrifugal force on the body in units of the earth's gravity.

H

hemifacial Involving half of the face divided at a vertical line at midface.

Hippocratic oath Ethical code attributed to the ancient Greek physician Hippocrates, adopted as a guide of conduct by those practicing medicine, the most important of which is "First do no harm."

I

incisional surgery Intervention that requires an incision, dissection, and repair.

indigenous population Original people inhabiting an area, as in the original inhabitants of far-North America in Alaska.

investigational new drug (IND) Authorization by the Food and Drug Administration (FDA) for an investigator to begin supervised study of a new drug employing human subjects.

in vivo Occurring in a living organism.

L

laminar flow Smooth air flow with no particle mixing.

lateral rectus Outward pulling muscle attached to the outer surface of each eyeball.

LD50 A dose that will kill 50 percent of laboratory animals treated.

lethal An action or substance that can kill.

lingual Relating to the tongue.

local anesthesia Numbing a small area with a topically applied or injected agent.

locked in Action or activity that is unwavering.

lysergic acid (LSD) A substance first used by private citizens as a mind-altering drug, producing a hallucinatory experience. After a series of bad experiences, including scientific experiments, it was made a Category I drug and illegal for any use outside of research. A branch of the Central Intelligence Agency (CIA) explored its use for information gathering, leading to the death of one victim.

M

Manhattan Project The code name for the World War II secret project to develop the atomic bomb.

masseter muscle A large muscle on either side of the face that supports the jaw and aids in chewing. Enlargement of this muscle can cause an unattractive widening of the lower face.

micrometer One millionth of a meter.

migraine Severe recurring headache that is disabling.

milliliter One thousandth of a liter.

molecule A group of atoms bonded together, representing the smallest fundamental unit of a chemical compound that can take part in a chemical reaction.

monomania Single-mindedly sticking to a single project, activity, or idea.

Monticello Thomas Jefferson's home in Virginia.

muckraker A person who digs up the dirt about someone or something and spreads the word.

myoclonus Repeated arrhythmic jerky movement of the trunk and limbs.

N

nanogram A billionth of a gram.

National Institutes of Health (NIH) Primary agency of the US government responsible for biomedical and public health research.

nerve A structure that delivers sensation to the brain and impulses to muscles and organs.

neuromuscular junction This is where the nerve impulse meets the muscle receptors to initiate contraction.

neurophysiologist A scientist who studies the function of the nervous system.

neurotoxin A biological substance that alters the structure or function of the nervous system.

normal saline A prescription medicine used for fluid and electrolyte replenishment. When sterile, suitable for intravenous administration and can be mixed with other agents.

O

Oculinum Brand name for botulinum toxin type A, later called Botox.

off the chart Having a bigger impact than anyone expected.

Office of Strategic Services (OSS) A governmental body headed by William Donovan beginning in 1943 with the charge of managing information (and disinformation) in support of the war effort. It was the forerunner of the present CIA.

orphan drug A drug that is useful but has a small market, making it eligible for lower FDA administrative costs and a longer period of exclusivity.

P

palette Roof of the mouth.

Paracelsus Said all things can be poison, it depends on the dose.

parasympathetic nervous system Helps run life-sustaining processes, like digestion, during times when you feel safe and relaxed; opposite of sympathetic nervous system.

Parkinson's disease A nervous system disorder affecting movement and causing tremors.

pH A figure expressing the acidity or alkalinity. A number of 7 is neutral, lower is acid, and higher is alkaline.

pharynx Throat comprising the upper part of the respiratory and digestive system.

poison A substance capable of causing illness or death.

primate Humans are primates. This class includes a diverse group of some two hundred species. Monkeys and apes are primates with many features in common with humans.

probiotic A combination of good bacteria and yeast that aids health and digestion.

procerus A facial muscle that connects the nasal bones and eyebrows.

prussic acid Hydrocyanic acid or cyanide, a highly lethal poison.

R

radiopharmacist A pharmacist who deals with special compounds and has practice following strict medical and government guidelines.

restless leg syndrome A nearly irresistible urge to move the legs.

S

Salmonella A bacterium that is a common cause of food poisoning.

saxitoxin Deadly toxin produced by shellfish.

smooth muscle Attached to organs and other structures not under voluntary control.

Space Race Competition between the Soviet Union and the United States, beginning in the late 1950s and continuing until 1975 when the two countries began to cooperate with space exploration.

Spanish-American War It took place in 1898, ending the Spanish colonial era in North America. Three thousand American soldiers died but most deaths were attributed to illness, including yellow fever, typhoid, and possibly botulism poisoning.

Special Operations Division (SOD) Part of the CIA responsible for paramilitary and covert activities, or "dirty tricks."

spore A cell that starts with or later develops a protective mechanism that can resist adverse environmental conditions.

squint Abnormal alignment of the eyes (strabismus).

Staphylococcus aureus A common bacterium that is the leading cause of skin and soft tissue infection.

strabismus Abnormal alignment of the eyes (squint).

Streptococcus pneumoniae A bacterium that is a common cause of respiratory infection.

striated muscle Aligned in bundles, they attach to the skeleton by tendon and are under control of the voluntary system.

Swabian Relating to the medieval German duchy of Swabia.

Swiss army knife This descriptive term is based on the example of the versatile, multifunction and highly useful Swiss army knife. The term is used to describe a thing or activity that is especially useful and versatile, often unexpectedly so.

sympathetic nervous system Responds when body is stressed, in danger, or physically active. This results in increased heart rate, slowed digestion, more efficient breathing, and dilated pupils. It is the opposite of the parasympathetic system.

synaptic vesicle Stores and releases a neurotransmitter.

T

Teflon A patented nonstick resin.

toxic Something that is harmful unpleasant or poisonous.

toxin A poison or venom of plant or animal origin that causes a response in a host.

toxoid A weakened toxin that induces an immune response in the body, especially the production of antibodies but does not cause illness.

trapezius A large muscle moving the back of the head and shoulder blades.

tremor Involuntary quivering movement.

U

U-2 plane A single-seat, high-altitude jet aircraft flown by the United States for intelligence gathering, surveillance, and reconnaissance. The term became synonymous with information gathering via filming from the air.

uremia This diagnosis of raised urea in the blood from reduced kidney function was affixed at the time because the attending physician was not sure of the cause of death and did not want to pursue further investigation. He chose this because of a prior diagnosis of kidney disease.

V

vaccine A substance used to stimulate the production of antibodies and provide immunity against one or several diseases.

VJ Day August 15, 1945, when Japan quit fighting in World War II.

Notes

Author's Note

1. Angeles R. Bort-Martí, Fiona J. Rowe, Laura Ruiz Sifre, Sueko M. Ng, Sylvia Bort-Martí, and Vicente Ruiz Garcia, "Botulinum Toxin for the Treatment of Strabismus," *The Cochrane Database of Systematic Reviews* 3, no. 3 (2023), CD006499, https://doi.org/10.1002/14651858.CD006499.pub5. The use of botulinum toxin as an investigative and treatment modality for strabismus is well reported in the medical literature. However, it is unclear how effective it is in comparison with other treatment options for strabismus.

1. CLOSTRIDIUM BOTULINUM

1. Penelope Green, "Alan Scott, Doctor Behind the Medical Use of Botox, Dies at 89," *New York Times*, January 12, 2022, https://www.nytimes.com/2022/01/12/health/alan-scott-dead.html.

2. Frank J. Erbguth, "The Pretherapeutic History of Botulinum Toxin," in *Manual of Botulinum Toxin Therapy*, 2nd ed., eds. Daniel Truong, Dirk Dressler, Mark Hallett, and Christopher Zachary (Cambridge, UK: Cambridge University Press, 2014), 1–8; F. J. Erbguth, "From Poison to Remedy: The Chequered History of Botulinum Toxin," *Journal of Neural Transmission (Vienna)* 115 (2008): 459–65.

3. Stephen C. Carlson, "(Blood) Sausage Banned," rtPanel, September 21, 2004, http://hypotyposeis.org/weblog/2004/09/blood-sausages-banned.html.

4. Erbguth, "Pretherapeutic History," 1.

5. Ibid., 2.

6. *Encyclopedia Britannica*, s.v. "Justinus Andreas Christian Kerner," German poet spiritualist and writer, accessed February 3, 2023, https://www.britannica.com/biography/Justinus-Andreas-Christian-Kerner.

7. Anna Mary Howitt Watts, *The Pioneers of the Spiritual Reformation: Life and Works of Dr. Justinius Kerner Adapted from the German; William Howitt and His Work for Spiritualism; Biographical Sketches* (London: The Psychological Press Association, 1883), http://iapsop.com/ssoc/1883__watts___life_and_work_of_justinus_kerner.pdf.

8. Published in *Graham's Magazine*, "The Wanderer in the Sawmill," XXXII, no. 2 (February 1848), https://fourteenlines.blog/tag/a-poets-solace-by-justinus-kerner/.

9. Justinus Kerner devised an inkblot process that was the precursor of the Rorschach test. John Foster, "The Inkblot and Popular Culture," Design Observer, April 28, 2013, https://designobserver.com/feature/the-inkblot-and-popular-culture/37853.

10. "That the peculiar work of blending the revelations . . . combined with additional confirmatory facts, before the world, in a strangely novel and romantic form, was reserved for Justinus Kerner." Anna Mary Howitt, "The Pioneers of the Spiritual Reformation. Life and Works of Justinus Kerner (Adapted from the German.) William Howitt and His Work for Spiritualism. Biographical Sketches," accessed February 3, 2023, https://archive.org/stream/pioneersofspiritoohowi/pioneersofspiritoohowi_djvu.txt.

11. Erbguth, "Pretherapeutic History," 2.

12. Rebecca Kreston, "The Bad Sausage & the Discovery of Botulism," *Discover*, July 31, 2016, https://www.discovermagazine.com/health/the-bad-sausage-and-the-discovery-of -botulism.

13. Ibid.

2. The World's Deadliest Poison

1. Ron Sender, Shai Fuchs, and Ron Milo, "Revised Estimates for the Number of Human and Bacteria Cells in the Body," *PLoS Biology* 14, no. 8 (2016): e1002533, https://doi .org/10.1371/journal.pbio.1002533.

2. Our bodies consist of trillions of microorganisms (also called microbiota or microbes) of thousands of different species, including bacteria that are good and potentially bad. "The Microbiome," The Nutrition Source, accessed February 3, 2023, https://www .hsph.harvard.edu/nutritionsource/microbiome/.

3. O. P. Kreyden, M. L. Geiges, R. Böni, and G. Burg, "Botulinum Toxin: From Poison to Drug. A Historical Review," *Hautarzt* 51, no. 10 (2000): 733–37, https://doi.org/10.1007 /s001050051206.

4. Catherine Offord, "Identifying a Killer, 1895," *The Scientist*, July 1, 2021, https:// www.the-scientist.com/foundations/identifying-a-killer-1895-68861.

5. William Bynum, "Robert Koch: How He Identified One of the 19th Century's Biggest Killers," *BBC Science Focus*, April 8, 2020, https://www.sciencefocus.com/the -human-body/robert-koch-how-he-identified-one-of-the-19th-centurys-biggest-killers/.

6. While there are said to be thirty thousand named species of bacteria, experts possibly using different numbers come up with varying numbers. There are a lot, including about one thousand different species, that live on/with humans. Daniel Dykhuizen, "Species Numbers in Bacteria," *Proceedings of the California Academy of Sciences* 56, no. 6, Suppl. 1 (2005): 62–71, https://www.ncbi.nlm.nih.gov/pmc/articles/PMC3160642 /#:~:text=How%20Many%20Named%20Species%20of,amplifying%20ribosomal%20 genes%20and%20sequencing.

7. Aman Tiwari and Shivaraj Nagalli, "Clostridium Botulinum," StatPearls [Internet], last updated August 8, 2022, https://www.ncbi.nlm.nih.gov/books/NBK553081/.

8. Botulinum toxin interferes with neural transmission by blocking the release of acetylcholine at the nerve ending. P. K. Nigam and Anjana Nigam, "Botulinum Toxin," *Indian Journal of Dermatology* 55, no. 1 (2010): 8–14, https://www.ncbi.nlm.nih.gov/pmc /articles/PMC2856357/.

9. Kate M. Cronan, "Infant Botulism," Nemours KidsHealth, February 2020, https://kidshealth.org/en/parents/botulism.html.

10. "The 6 Rules of FATTOM," Unilever Food Solutions, accessed February 3, 2023, https://www.unileverfoodsolutions.com.my/en/chef-inspiration/food-safety/the-6-rules-of-fattom.html.

11. Iain A. Jeffery and Shahnawaz Karim, "Botulism," StatPearls [Internet], last update July 18, 2022, https://www.ncbi.nlm.nih.gov/books/NBK459273/.

12. Frank J. Erbguth, "The Pretherapeutic History of Botulinum Toxin," in *Manual of Botulinum Toxin Therapy*, 2nd ed., eds. Daniel Truong, Dirk Dressler, Mark Hallett, and Christopher Zachary (Cambridge, UK: Cambridge University Press, 2014), 4.

13. Botox has a wide margin of safety. Ornella Rossetto and Cesare Montecucco, "Tables of Toxicity of Botulinum and Tetanus Neurotoxins," *Toxins* 11, no. 12 (2019): 686, https://doi.org/10.3390/toxins11120686.

14. *Encyclopedia Britannica*, s.v. "Paracelsus," German-Swiss physician, accessed February 3, 2023, https://www.britannica.com/biography/Paracelsus.

3. The Canning Industry

1. Nicolas-François Appert (born c. 1749, died June 3, 1841), French chef, confectioner, and distiller who invented the method of preserving food by enclosing it in a hermetically sealed container. *Encyclopedia Britannica*, s.v. "Nicolas Appert," French chef, accessed February 3, 2023, https://www.britannica.com/biography/Nicolas-Appert.

2. This saying, which attests to the importance of forces being well-provisioned, has been attributed to both Napoleon and Frederick the Great. "An Army Marches on Its Stomach," Oxford Reference, accessed February 3, 2023, https://www.oxfordreference.com/view/10.1093/oi/authority.20110803095425331.

3. Martin H. Stack, "Canning Industry," Encyclopedia.com, accessed October 15, 2021, https://www.encyclopedia.com/history/dictionaries-thesauruses-pictures-and-press-releases/canning-industry.

4. "The Assassination of President William McKinley," History.com, accessed February 3, 2023, https://www.history.com/news/the-assassination-of-president-william-mckinley.

5. Jonathan Rees, "The Chemistry of Fear: Harvey Wiley's Fight for Pure Food," Johns Hopkins University Press, July 8, 2021, https://www.press.jhu.edu/newsroom/chemistry-fear-harvey-wileys-fight-pure-food.

6. Shahan Russell, "Unexpected Consequences—How the Spanish-American War Improved American Food," War History Online, December 16, 2017, https://www.warhistoryonline.com/instant-articles/spanish-american-war-american-food.html?chrome=1.

7. Anthony Gaughan and Peter Barton Hutt, "Harvey Wiley, Theodore Roosevelt, and the Federal Regulation of Food and Drug," LEDA at Harvard Law School, Winter 2004, https://dash.harvard.edu/bitstream/handle/1/8852144/Gaughan.html.

8. In 1850, medical diagnostics were rudimentary, autopsies were rare, and reliable data were scarce. Stephen Berry and Tracy L. Barnett, "The Graveyard of Old Diseases," CSI: *Dixie*, May 7, 2019, https://csidixie.org/numbers/mortality-census/graveyard-old-diseases.

9. Safe processing of canned foods involves correct time, temperature, and pressure. Martha Zepp, "Time, Temperature, Pressure in Canning Foods," PennState Extension, updated November 3, 2020, https://extension.psu.edu/time-temperature-pressure-in -canning-foods.

4. An Outbreak in the United States

1. Anna Zeide, "The Botulism Outbreak That Gave Rise to America's Food Safety System," *Smithsonian*, August 3, 2018, https://www.smithsonianmag.com/history/botulism -outbreak-gave-rise-americas-food-safety-system-180969868/.

2. Dan Flynn, "Canned Ripe California Olives Spread Botulism in 1919," *Food Safety News*, March 19, 2012, https://www.foodsafetynews.com/2012/03/canned-ripe-california -olives-spread-botulism-in-1919/.

3. Shane Hoover, "High Society, Bad Olives and a Window into Alliance's Past," *The Repository*, October 25, 2015, https://www.cantonrep.com/story/news/local/2015/10/25 /high-society-bad-olives-window/33209414007/.

4. "Give Dr. Armstrong a mouse and a syringe, and he can do research." Edward A. Beeman, "Charles Armstrong, M.D.: A Biography," The Tribune School, 2007, https:// www.tribuneschoolchd.com/uploads/tms/files/1595165269-charles-armstrong-m-d--a -biography-pdfdrive-com-.pdf.

5. Dan Flynn, "Canned Ripe California Olives Spread Botulism in 1919," *Food Safety News*, March 19, 2012, https://www.foodsafetynews.com/2012/03/canned-ripe-california -olives-spread-botulism-in-1919/.

6. James Harvey Young, "Botulism and the Ripe Olive Scare of 1919–1920," *Bulletin of the History of Medicine* 50, no. 3 (Fall 1976): 372–91.

7. Oil for Life as Thomas Jefferson put it, "The olive tree is surely the richest gift of heaven." "Oil for Life," *1843 magazine, The Economist*, May 9, 2006, https://www .economist.com/news/2006/05/09/oil-for-life.

8. The "father" of black olives and Freda Ehmann "mother" of California ripe olives. Frederic T. Bioletti, "Frederic T. Bioletti Papers," Online Archive of California, 1881–1935, https://oac.cdlib.org/findaid/ark:/13030/kt1h4nd9oz/entire_text/.

9. Charles Richter and John S. Emrich, "Karl F. Meyer: The Renaissance Immunologist," American Association of Immunologists, June/July 2018, pp. 22–27, https://www .aai.org/About/History/History-Articles-Keep-for-Hierarchy/Karl-F-Meyer-The -Renaissance-Immunologist.

10. J. Russell Esty, "Control of the Processing of Canned Foods in California," *American Journal of Public Health*, accessed February 3, 2023, https://ajph.aphapublications.org /doi/pdf/10.2105/AJPH.25.2.165.

5. A Rare and Deadly Disease

1. This story is based on the following case report: Matthias Gerhard Vossen, Klaus-Bernhard Gattringer, Judith Wenisch, Neda Khalifeh, Maria Koreny, Verena Spertini, Franz Allerberger, et al., "The First Case(s) of Botulism in Vienna in 21 Years: A Case Report," *Case Reports in Infectious Disease* (2012): 438989, https://doi.org/10.1155/2012 /438989.

2. Agam K. Rao, Jeremy Sobel, Kevin Chatham-Stephens, and Carolina Luquez, "Clinical Guidelines for Diagnosis and Treatment of Botulism, 2021," *Recommendations and Reports* 70, no. 2 (2021): 1–30, https://www.cdc.gov/mmwr/volumes/70/rr/rr7002a1 .htm.

3. Ibid.

4. Botulism in poultry is known as "limberneck." Rachel, "Botulism in Chickens—Signs, Symptoms and Prevention," Dine a Chook, February 25, 2019, https://www .dineachook.com.au/blog/botulism-in-chickens-signs-symptoms-and-prevention/.

6. World War II Sets the Stage

1. "Roosevelt and Churchill: A Friendship That Saved the World," National Park Service, accessed February 3, 2023, https://www.nps.gov/articles/fdrww2.htm.

2. "America First and WWII," Charles Lindbergh House and Museum, accessed February 3, 2023, https://www.mnhs.org/lindbergh/learn/controversies.

3. "'Wild Bill' Donovan and the Origin of the OSS," National Park Service, accessed February 3, 2023, https://www.nps.gov/articles/wild-bill-donovan-and-the-origins-of -the-oss.htm.

4. "Destroyers for Bases Agreement, September 2, 1940," Robert H. Jackson Center, September 2, 2015, https://www.roberthjackson.org/article/destroyers-for-bases -agreement-september-2-1940/.

5. Richard Gid Powers, "Undercover Rivalries," *Washington Post*, October 23, 1994, https://www.washingtonpost.com/archive/entertainment/books/1994/10/23/undercover -rivalries/5c46a3ed-b6f5-4dde-ba67-bf208a7abbef/.

6. Brian Balmer, "Biological Warfare: The Threat in Historical Perspective," *Medicine, Conflict and Survival* 18, no. 2 (April–June 2002): 120–37, https://www.jstor.org/stable /45352052.

7. "Fort Detrick: A Timeline," Fort Detrick Alliance, accessed February 3, 2023, https://www.fortdetrickalliance.org/history.html.

7. Camp Detrick—US Army Biological Warfare Laboratories

1. Robert Farley and Lori Robertson, "Hitler and Chemical Weapons," FactCheck Posts, April 12, 2017, https://www.factcheck.org/2017/04/hitler-chemical-weapons/.

2. "The Terrifying German 'Revenge Weapons' of the Second World War," Imperial War Museums, accessed February 3, 2023, https://www.iwm.org.uk/history/the -terrifying-german-revenge-weapons-of-the-second-world-war.

3. "Biological Weapons," GlobalSecurity.org, accessed February 6, 2023, https://www .globalsecurity.org/wmd/systems/bw.htm.

4. "Manhattan Project," History.com, updated April 19, 2022, https://www.history .com/topics/world-war-ii/the-manhattan-project.

5. George W. Merck, "Report to the Secretary of War by Mr. George W. Merck, Special Consultant for Biological Warfare," National Academy of Sciences, January 3, 1945, http://www.nasonline.org/about-nas/history/archives/collections/organized-collections /1945merckreport.pdf.

6. Fort Detrick USAG, "#ThrowbackThursday," Facebook, March 20, 2014, https://www.facebook.com/photo/?fbid=629238880484612&set=throwbackthursdaytbt-the-black-maria-was-the-first-laboratory-facility-built-to-.

7. HistoryNet Staff, "Dr. Ira Baldwin: Biological Weapons Pioneer," HistoryNet, June 12, 2006, https://www.historynet.com/dr-ira-baldwin-biological-weapons-pioneer/.

8. Carl Lamanna, "The Most Poisonous Poison: What Do We Know about the Toxin of Botulism? What Are the Problems to Be Solved?," *Science* 130, no. 3378 (1959): 763–72, https://www.science.org/doi/10.1126/science.130.3378.763.

9. John D. Hall, "Arthur C. Guyton, MD 1919–2003," *Circulation* 107, no. 24 (2003): 2990–92, https://www.ahajournals.org/doi/10.1161/01.CIR.0000080480.62058.4A.

10. E. J. Schantz, "Oral History Interview with Edward J. Schantz [sound recording]," ArchiveGrid, 1997, https://researchworks.oclc.org/archivegrid/data/526697253.

11. Eric Johnson, personal communication, November 2021.

8. Fort Detrick and the CIA

1. "It was signed by Ira Baldwin, assistant dean of the College of Agriculture." Stephen Kinzer, *Poisoner in Chief: Sidney Gottlieb and the CIA Search for Mind Control* (New York: Henry Holt & Co., 2019), 6.

2. Kinzer, *Poisoner in Chief*, 50.

3. Ibid., 38.

4. Ibid., 13.

5. LSD is listed as class I with no medical use with high potential for addiction. Kristopher Hooks, "Marijuana, LSD and the Story of Other Schedule 1 Drugs," abc10, May 7, 2017, https://www.abc10.com/article/news/marijuana-lsd-and-the-story-of-other-schedule-1-drugs/103-436904118.

6. S. J. Novak, "LSD before Leary, Sidney Cohen's Critique of 1950s Psychedelic Drug Research," March 1997, https://pubmed.ncbi.nlm.nih.gov/9154737.

7. "Family in LSD Case Gets Ford Apology," *New York Times*, July 22, 1975, 1, https://www.nytimes.com/1975/07/22/archives/family-in-lsd-case-gets-ford-apology-family-in-lsd-death-case-gets.html.

8. Danielle E. Gaines, "Lawsuit by Family of Drugged Detrick Employee Dismissed," *Frederick News-Post*, July 18, 2013, https://www.fredericknewspost.com/news/crime_and_justice/article_8705f623-edfd-59b0-9e04-548b15a2c423.html?TNNoMobile.

9. Kinzer, *Poisoner in Chief*, 174.

10. "U-2 Overflights and the Capture of Francis Gary Powers, 1960," Office of the Historian, Foreign Service Institute, accessed February 6, 2023, https://history.state.gov/milestones/1953-1960/u2-incident.

11. Kinzer, *Poisoner in Chief*, 171.

12. Ibid., 175.

13. Improved U2s still flying. Emma Helfrich and Tyler Rogoway, "The U-2 Dragon Lady Finally Says Goodbye to Film Cameras at Beale AFB," *The Drive*, July 1, 2022, https://www.thedrive.com/the-war-zone/beale-air-force-base-finally-says-goodbye-to-film-for-its-u-2-spy-planes.

14. Lumumba dies at firing squad: *Encyclopedia Britannica*, s.v. "How Did Patrice Lumumba Die?," accessed February 3, 2023, https://www.britannica.com/story/how-did-patrice-lumumba-die.

15. Alexander Smith, "Fidel Castro: The CIA's 7 Most Bizarre Assassination Attempts," *NBC News*, November 28, 2016, https://www.nbcnews.com/storyline/fidel-castros-death/fidel-castro-cia-s-7-most-bizarre-assassination-attempts-n688951.

16. Schantz testimony: United States Senate, "U.S. Senate, Select Committee to Study Governmental Operations with Respect to Intelligence Activities," Assassination Archive and Research Center, Washington, DC, Thursday, September 18, 1975, 139–59, https://www.aarclibrary.org/publib/church/reports/vol1/pdf/ChurchV1_5_Schantz.pdf.

9. The Government Steps In

1. Jonathan B. Tucker and Erin R. Mahan, *President Nixon's Decision to Renounce the U.S. Offensive Biological Weapons Program* (Washington, DC: National Defense University Press, 2009), https://ndupress.ndu.edu/Portals/68/Documents/casestudies/CSWMD_CaseStudy-1.pdf.

2. Allergan obtains FDA approval for new botulinum toxin culture. "Allergan Receives FDA Approval for First-of-Its-Kind, Fully *In Vitro*, Cell-Based Assay for BOTOX® and BOTOX® Cosmetic (onabotulinumtoxinA)," *Eastern Daylight Time* (Business Wire), June 24, 2011, https://www.businesswire.com/news/home/20110624005918/en/Allergan-Receives-FDA-Approval-for-First-of-Its-Kind-Fully-in-vitro-Cell-Based-Assay-for-BOTOX%C2%AE-and-BOTOX%C2%AE-Cosmetic-onabotulinumtoxinA.

3. United States Congress Senate Select Committee, *Hearings before the Select Committee to Study Governmental Operations with Respect to Intelligence Activities of the United States Senate: Ninety-fourth Congress, First Session. Volume 1: Unauthorized Storage of Toxic Agents* (Washington, DC: US Government Printing Office, 1976), https://www.intelligence.senate.gov/sites/default/files/94intelligence_activities_I.pdf.

4. Ibid.

5. Ibid.

10. Edward Schantz Testifies

1. United States Senate, "U.S. Senate, Select Committee to Study Governmental Operations with Respect to Intelligence Activities," Assassination Archive and Research Center, Washington, DC, Thursday, September 18, 1975, 139–59, https://www.aarclibrary.org/publib/church/reports/vol1/pdf/ChurchV1_5_Schantz.pdf.

2. Ibid., 139.

3. Ibid., 140.

4. Ibid.

5. Ibid., 141.

6. Ibid., 148.

7. Ibid., 141.

8. Ibid., 153.

9. Ibid., 144.

10. Ibid., 158.

11. Back in Madison

1. Jeremy Pearce, "Edward J. Schantz, Pioneering Researcher of Toxins, Including Botox, Dies at 96," *New York Times*, May 4, 2005, https://www.nytimes.com/2005/05/04/us/edward-j-schantz-pioneering-researcher-of-toxins-including-botox-dies-at.html.

2. Eric Johnson, personal communication, November 2021.

3. Daniel Drachman, personal communication, October 2021.

4. Eric Johnson, personal communication, November 2021.

5. Vernon Brooks, "Vernon B. Brooks," in *The History of Neuroscience in Autobiography*, vol. 3, ed. Larry R. Squire (San Diego, CA: Academic Press, 2001), 82n1, https://www.sfn.org/-/media/SfN/Documents/TheHistoryofNeuroscience/Volume-3/c3.pdf.

6. World War II Research, 1944–1946. A. Edward Maumenee, MD, *Ophthalmology*. Oral History Series, A Link with Our Past, an oral history conducted in 1990 by Sally Smith Hughes, Regional Oral History Office, University of California, Berkeley, in cooperation with The Foundation of the American Academy of Ophthalmology, p. 46. Copyright 1994. "Oral Histories," American Academy of Ophthalmology, accessed February 4, 2023, https://www.aao.org/oral-histories.

7. Alan B. Scott, personal communication, November 2021.

8. D. B. Drachman, ed., *Johns Hopkins Neurology: Half a Century of Innovation* (Baltimore, MD: Johns Hopkins Department of Neurology, The Johns Hopkins University and The Johns Hopkins Health System Corporation, Johns Hopkins University Press, 2019), 36.

9. D. B. Drachman, "Atrophy of Skeletal Muscle in Chick Embryos Treated with Botulinum Toxin," *Science* 145, no. 3633 (1964): 719–21.

10. Drachman, *Half a Century*, 36.

12. Dr. Alan B. Scott

1. "The Forty Niners," Library of Congress, accessed February 4, 2023, https://www.loc.gov/collections/california-first-person-narratives/articles-and-essays/early-california-history/forty-niners/#:~:text=Not%20everyone%20who%20came%20to,miners%20with%20goods%20and%20services.

2. Alan B. Scott, personal communication, October and November 2021. This includes all other references to Scott comments in quotation marks.

3. Charles Richter and John S. Emrich, "Karl F. Meyer: The Renaissance Immunologist," American Association of Immunologists, June/July 2018, pp. 22–27, https://www.aai.org/About/History/History-Articles-Keep-for-Hierarchy/Karl-F-Meyer-The-Renaissance-Immunologist.

4. Alan B. Scott, personal communication, October 2021.

13. Progress in the Lab

1. Alan Scott, personal communication, November 2021.

2. Smith-Kettlewell, "About SKERI," accessed February 4, 2023, https://www.ski.org.

3. Alan Scott, personal communication, October 2021.

4. Elbert Magoon, personal communication, March 2022.

14. First Injection in a Primate

1. Daniel B. Drachman, ed., *Johns Hopkins Neurology: Half a Century of Innovation* (Baltimore, MD: Johns Hopkins Department of Neurology, The Johns Hopkins University and The Johns Hopkins Health System Corporation, Johns Hopkins University Press, 2019), 36.

2. Alan B. Scott, personal communication, October 2021.

3. Drachman, *Half a Century*, 1.

4. A. B. Scott, A. L. Rosenbaum, and C. C. Collins, "Pharmacologic Weakening of Extraocular Muscles," *Investigative Ophthalmology* 12 (1973): 924–27.

5. "Who We Are," The Association for Research in Vision and Ophthalmology, accessed February 4, 2023, https://www.arvo.org/About/who-we-are.

6. Scott, Rosenbaum, and Collins, "Pharmacologic Weakening of Extraocular Muscles," 927.

7. Chuck McCutcheon, "The Creator of Botox Never Cared about Wrinkles," *Scientific American* (Guest Blog), November 3, 2016, https://blogs.scientificamerican.com/guest-blog/the-creator-of-botox-never-cared-about-wrinkles/.

8. Jean D. Carruthers, "Beneath the Surface of Botox," Filmed October 21, 2012, at TEDxVancouver, Vancouver, British Columbia, video, 17:07, https://www.youtube.com/watch?v=cuEZ8I_lZeo.

9. Alan B. Scott, personal communication, November 2021.

15. First Injection in a Human

1. The Pure Food and Drug Act was the FDA's founding statute created in response to scandals in the meatpacking industry widely exposed in Upton Sinclair's book, the jungle. "Pure Food and Drug Act," ScienceDirect, accessed February 4, 2023, https://www.sciencedirect.com/topics/agricultural-and-biological-sciences/pure-food-and-drug-act.

2. United States Senate, "U.S. Senate, Select Committee to Study Governmental Operations with Respect to Intelligence Activities," Assassination Archive and Research Center, Washington, DC, Thursday, September 18, 1975, 141, https://www.aarclibrary.org/publib/church/reports/vol1/pdf/ChurchV1_5_Schantz.pdf.

3. Under FDA regulations, an institutional review board is a group that has been formally designated to review and monitor biomedical research involving human subjects. "Institutional Review Boards (IRBs) and Protection of Human Subjects in Clinical Trials," US Food and Drug Administration, accessed February 4, 2023, https://www.fda.gov/about-fda/center-drug-evaluation-and-research-cder/institutional-review-boards-irbs-and-protection-human-subjects-clinical-trials.

4. "FDA Drug Approval Process," US Food and Drug Administration, accessed February 4, 2024, https://www.fda.gov/media/82381/download.

5. A conservative estimate of the cost of conducting trials for a new drug is nearly $70 million. Patricio Ledesma, "How Much Does a Clinical Trial Cost?," Sofpromed, January 2, 2020, https://www.sofpromed.com/how-much-does-a-clinical-trial-cost.

6. Some drug approval costs are in the billions. Michael Schlander, Karla Hernandez-Villafuerte, Chih-Yuan Cheng, Jorge Mestre-Ferrandiz, and Michael Baumann, "How Much Does It Cost to Research and Develop a New Drug? A Systematic Review and

Assessment," *PharmacoEconomics* 39 (2021): 1243–69, https://link.springer.com/article/10
.1007/s40273-021-01065-y.

7. "Alan Scott, MD: The Story of Botox in His Own Words," The Barkan Society, accessed February 4, 2023, https://barkansociety.com/alan-scott-the-story-of-botox-in-his
-own-words/.

8. Alan B. Scott, "Botulinum Toxin Injection of Eye Muscles to Correct Strabismus,"
Transactions of the American Ophthalmological Society 79 (1981): 734–69, https://www
.ncbi.nlm.nih.gov/pmc/articles/PMC1312202/.

9. Ibid.

10. Elbert Magoon, personal communication, May 2022.

11. Scott, "Botulinum Toxin Injection."

12. Alan Scott, personal communication, October 2021.

16. Joining the Team

1. Personal communication with Alan B. Scott, November 2021.

2. G. K. vonNoorden, ed., *The History of Strabismology* (Belgium: J. P. Wayenborgh,
2018), 152.

3. E. M. Helveston and A. E. Pogrebniak, "Treatment of Acquired Nystagmus with
Botulinum A Toxin," *American Journal of Ophthalmology* 106, no. 5 (1988): 584–86.

17. Manufacturing Begins

1. Biological require a regulated manufacturing process for FDA approval. "Biologics License Applications (BLA) Process (CBER)," US Food and Drug Administration,
January 27, 2021, https://www.fda.gov/vaccines-blood-biologics/development-approval-
process-cber/biologics-license-applications-bla-process-cber.

2. Alan B. Scott, personal communication, October 2021.

3. Dennis Honeychurch, personal communication, October 2021.

4. Botox is useful for both cosmetics and therapeutics. John Infanti, "The Surprising
Uses of Botox," Penn Medicine, July 25, 2018, https://www.pennmedicine.org/news/news
-blog/2018/july/the-surprising-uses-of-botox.

5. Bupivacaine injection remodels muscles and corrects comitant strabismus. Joel M.
Miller, Alan B. Scott, Kenneth K. Danth, Dirk Strasser, and Mona Sane, "Bupivacaine Injection Remodels Extraocular Muscles and Corrects Comitant Strabismus," *Ophthalmology* 120, no. 12 (2013): 2733–40, https://www.aaojournal.org/article/S0161-6420(13)00494-6
/fulltext.

6. Alexandra Sifferlin, "Botox: The Drug That's Treating Everything," *Time*, January
5, 2017, https://time.com/magazine/us/4623396/january-16th-2017-vol-189-no-3-u-s/.

18. Marketing and Selling a New Drug

1. Alan B. Scott comments in the foreword to this book: Joseph Jankovic, Alberto
Albanese, M. Zouhair Atassi, J. Oliver Dolly, Mark Hallett, and Nathaniel H. Mayer,
Botulinum Toxin: Therapeutic Clinical Practice and Science (Philadelphia, PA: Saunders
an imprint by Elsevier, 2009), xii.

2. Leah Nylen, "ITC to Decide Botox Trade Secret Battle," *Politico*, November 18,
2020, https://www.politico.com/news/2020/11/18/jeaveau-botox-us-ban-437823#:~:text

=A%20fight%20at%20the%20International,for%20the%20next%2010%20years.&text
=If%20Abbvie's%20Allergan%20gets%20its,for%20the%20next%2010%20years.

Scott Alan B, Magoon Elbert H, McNeer Keith W, Stager, D,. Botulinum Treatment of Strabismus In Children Tr. Am. Ophth. Soc. Vol LXXXVII, 1989, pp. 174-184.

3. Sports drink dollar sales in the United States from 2013 to 2018, by brand. "Sports Drink Sales in U.S. Convenience Stores (C-Stores) in 2021, by Brand," Statista, April 2022, https://www.statista.com/statistics/408970/best-selling-sports-drink-brands-in-us-c -stores-based-on-dollar-sales/.

4. "Soaring Prices on Decades-old Drugs," Susan Collins, May 6, 2016, https://www .collins.senate.gov/newsroom/soaring-prices-decades-old-drugs.

5. Michael L. Schilsky, Eve A. Roberts, Sihoun Hahn, and Frederick Askari, "Costly Choices for Treating Wilson's Disease," *Hepatology* 61, no. 4 (2015): 1106–8.

6. Gemma Jones, "Court Throws Out Allergan's Patent Deal with Native American Tribe," *PMLiVE*, October 18, 2017, https://www.pmlive.com/pharma_news/court_throws _out_allergans_patent_deal_with_native_american_tribe_1208729.

7. Nathan Bomey, "Humira Maker AbbVie to Acquire Botox Maker Allergan for $63 Billion," *USA Today*, June 25, 2019, https://www.usatoday.com/story/money/2019/06/25 /abbvie-allergan-acquisition-merger/1556361001/.

8. Kevin Dunleavy, "Humira Rings Up $20.7B in 2021, but AbbVie Still Mum on Post-biosimilar Expectations," Fierce Pharma, February 2, 2022, https://www.fiercepharma .com/pharma/humira-rings-up-20-7-billion-sales-but-abbvie-still-mum-a-projection -for-2023-when-it-faces.

9. Mark Terry, "The Median Drug Development Cost is $985 Million, According to New Study," BioSpace, March 4, 2020, https://www.biospace.com/article/median-cost-of -bringing-a-new-drug-to-market-985-million/.

10. Katie Thomas, "Severe Eczema Drug Is Approved by F.D.A.: Price Tag Is $37,000 a Year," *New York Times*, March 28, 2017, https://www.nytimes.com/2017/03/28/health /drug-prices-fda-eczema-skin-disease.html.

11. "New Estimate Puts Cost to Develop a New Drug at $1B," Biotechnology Community, March 20, 2020, https://biotechnologycommunity.com/md_news/new-estimate -puts-cost-to-develop-a-new-drug-at-1b/.

12. Olivier J. Wouters, Martin McKee, and Jeroen Luyten, "Estimated Research and Development Investment Needed to Bring a New Medicine to Market, 2009–2018," *JAMA* 323, no. 9 (2020): 844–53, https://pubmed.ncbi.nlm.nih.gov/32125404/.

13. "Orphan Drug," National Cancer Institute, accessed February 5, 2023, https:// cancer.gov/publications/dictionaries/cancer-terms/def/orphan-drug; "Search Orphan Drug Designations and Approvals," US Food and Drug Administration, accessed February 5, 2023, https://www.accessdata.fda.gov/scripts/opdlisting/oopd/detailedIndex.cfm ?cfgridkey=483.

19. Botox and Beauty

1. Jean D. Carruthers, "Beneath the Surface of Botox: Dr. Jean Carruthers at TEDx Vancouver," streamed live on February 6, 2013, YouTube video, 00:17:07, https://www .youtube.com/watch?v=cuEZ8I_lZeo.

2. Alistair Carruthers and Jean Carruthers, eds., *Botulinum Toxin: Procedures in Cosmetic Dermatology*, 4th ed. (Toronto, ON: Elsevier, 2018), preface.

3. Personal communication Jean Carruthers, January 2022.

20. Dermatology Opens the Floodgates

1. William Hanke, personal communication, November 2022.

2. Cosmetic Dermatologic Surgery Fellowship Program, "Frequently Asked Questions FAQs," accessed February 6, 2023, https://www.asds.net/Portals/0/PDF/cosmetic-accreditation-fellowship-faq.pdf.

3. "ASDS Reveals Annual Award Recipients at 2020: ASDS Virtual Annual Meeting," Medindia, October 12, 2020, https://www.medindia.net/health-press-release/asds-reveals-annual-award-recipients-at-2020-asds-virtual-annual-meeting-491898-1.htm.

4. Alistair Carruthers and Jean Carruthers, eds., *Botulinum Toxin: Procedures in Cosmetic Dermatology*, 4th ed. (Toronto, ON: Elsevier, 2018), preface.

5. Joseph Jankovic, Alberto Albanese, M. Zouhair Atassi, J. Oliver Dolly, Mark Hallett, and Nathaniel H. Mayer, *Botulinum Toxin: Therapeutic Clinical Practice and Science* (Philadelphia, PA: Saunders Elsevier, 2009), 324–38.

6. Heather Buschman, "Headline News: Botox Injections May Lessen Depression," UC San Diego Health, July 30, 2020, https://health.ucsd.edu/news/releases/Pages/2020-07-30-headline-news-botox-may-lessen-depression.aspx.

7. BTX can be safely used in the treatment of chronic pain where complications from drug treatment are a concern. Woo Seog Sim, "Application of Botulinum Toxin in Pain Management," *Korean Journal of Pain* 24, no. 1 (2011): 1–6, https://www.ncbi.nlm.nih.gov/pmc/articles/PMC3049971/.

21. Botox in Neurology

1. Andrew Blitzer, Mitchell F. Brin, and Celia F. Stewart, "Botulinum Toxin Management of Spasmodic Dysphonia (Laryngeal Dystonia): A 12-Year Experience in More Than 900 Patients†," *Laryngoscope* 108 (1998): 1435–41, https://doi.org/10.1097/00005537-199810000-00003.

2. "Neuron and Nerves," Vedantu, last updated February 4, 2023, https://www.vedantu.com/biology/neuron-and-nerves.

3. Kendra Cherry, "The Size of the Human Brain: Brain Weight, Brain Length, and Intelligence," Verywell Mind, last updated May 17, 2022, https://www.verywellmind.com/how-big-is-the-brain-2794888.

4. Tom Valeo, "New Brain-Imaging Techniques Help Diagnose Neurologic Conditions," *Brain&Life*, October/November 2013, https://www.brainandlife.org/articles/new-brain-imaging-techniques-provide-better-ways-to-diagnose-and.

5. Ibid.

6. Charenya Anandan and Joseph Jankovic, "Botulinum Toxin in Movement Disorders: An Update," *Toxins (Basel)* thirteen, no. 1 (2021): 42, https://doi.org/10.3390/toxins13010042.

7. Stephen D. Silberstein, "Botulinum Toxin in Headache Management," in *Botulinum Toxin: Therapeutic Clinical Practice and Science*, eds. Joseph Jankovic, Alberto

Albanese, M. Zouhair Atassi, J. Oliver Dolly, Mark Hallett, and Nathaniel H. Mayer (Philadelphia, PA: Saunders Elsevier, 2009), 214.

8. Millions suffer from migraine and disabling headaches. Rebecca Burch, Paul Rizzoli, and Elizabeth Loder, "The Prevalence and Impact of Migraine and Severe Headache in the United States: Figures and Trends from Government Health Studies," *Headache* 58, no. 4 (2018): 496–505, https://pubmed.ncbi.nlm.nih.gov/29527677/.

9. "Botulinum Toxin," *Medical Clinical Policy Bulletins*, Aetna, accessed February 6, 2023, http://www.aetna.com/cpb/medical/data/100_199/0113.html.

10. Allison Brashear, Mark F Gordon, Elie Elovic, V. Daniel Kassicieh, Christina Marciniak, Mai Do, Chia-Ho Lee, Stephen Jenkins, Catherine Turkel, and Botox Post-Stroke Spasticity Study Group, "Intramuscular Injection of Botulinum Toxin for the Treatment of Wrist and Finger Spasticity after a Stroke," *New England Journal of Medicine* 347, no. 6 (2002): 395–four hundred.

11. Personal communication, Christi George, December 2021.

22. THE LEGACY

1. Walter Isaacson, *The Code Breaker* (New York: Simon & Schuster, 2021), 475.

2. Jackie Lehmer, personal communication, October 2022.

APPENDIX 1

1. *Encyclopedia Britannica*, s.v. "Justinus Andreas Christian Kerner," accessed February 6, 2023, https://www.britannica.com/biography/Justinus-Andreas-Christian-Kerner.

2. Anna Mary Howitt, "The Pioneers of the Spiritual Reformation. Life and Works of Dr. Justinus Kerner (Adapted from the German.) William Howitt and His Work for Spiritualism. Biographical Sketches," accessed February 3, 2023, https://archive.org/stream/pioneersofspiritoohowi/pioneersofspiritoohowi_djvu.txt.

3. "The Wanderer in the Sawmill by Justinus Kerner (1786–1862)," translated by William Cullen Bryant, Fourteen Lines, accessed February 4, 2023, https://fourteenlines.blog/tag/the-wanderer-in-the-sawmill-by-justinus-kerner/.

APPENDIX 2

1. "Karl F. Meyer, D.V.M., Ph.D.," American Association of Immunologists, accessed February 6, 2023, https://www.aai.org/About/History/Past-Presidents-and-Officers/KarlFMeyer.

APPENDIX 3

1. *Mississippi Encyclopedia*, s.v. "Arthur C. Guyton," accessed February 6, 2023, https://mississippiencyclopedia.org/entries/arthur-c-guyton/.

2. Frank J. Lebeda, Michael Adler, and Zygmunt F. Dembek, "Yesterday and Today: The Impact of Research Conducted at Camp Detrick on Botulinum Toxin," *Military Medicine* 183, nos. 5–6 (May–June 2018): 85–95, https://doi.org/10.1093/milmed/usx047.

Index

Note: Page numbers in *italics* refer to illustrations.

California Pacific Medical Center, 83, 97–98, 99, 100
California State Prison, 85–86
Campbell Soup Company, 19
Camp Detrick (later Fort Detrick): and assassination plans, 53–54; biological weapons research at, 40, 42–47; and Church Committee hearings, 57–59, 65; and CIA, 40, 48–54, 55, 61; and government intervention, 55–58; Guyton's research at, 70; LSD research at, 49–50; Maumenee's work at, 68; saxitoxin (shellfish toxin) at, 45, 52–53, 57, 61–62; and Schantz's Senate testimony, 60; and suicide option for U-2 pilots, 51–53; and vaccines for botulinum toxin, 51
camptocormia (flexion of trunk), 149
Cannery Inspection Act (1925), 28
canning: advent of commercial, 21, 23; and conditions necessary for botulism, 21; and defense against botulism poisoning, 13; destruction of C. botulinum toxin in, 10, 73; development of commercial, 17, 18–19; home canning practices, 22, 29; origins of term, 18–19; and research on botulism, 73; and safe food practices, 19–22, 29, 44; transmission of spores to cans, 9
Carruthers, Alastair, 131, 132, 134, 141, 142
Carruthers, Jean, 131–37, 140–41, 142
Castro, Fidel, 53–54, 58
Centers for Disease Control and Prevention (CDC) Emergency Operations Center, 29
Central Intelligence Agency (CIA): assassination plots of, 53–54; biological/chemical weapons research of, 55; and Camp Detrick, 40, 49–54, 55, 61; and Church Committee hearings, 51, 53, 54, 57–59, 60–65; establishment of, 40; goals of, 40; and LSD research, 49–50; plans to deploy toxins exposed, 47; and Schantz's Senate testimony, 60; and suicide option for U-2 pilots, 51–53
cerebral palsy, 144, 156
cervical dystonia, 149, 156
Child, Paul and Julia, 39

Church, Frank, 57, 60–61, 63, 64–65
Church Committee hearings, 51, 53, 54, 57–59, 60–65
Churchill, Winston, 36
clinical trials for botulinum toxin: botulinum toxin needed for, 56; Carruthers' participation in, 133; commencement of, 156; costs associated with, 100, 129; data from, 120–21; donations requested for drugs in, 113, 115, 120, 129; and FDA oversight, 97, 100–101, 108; first phase of, 99–108; initial procedure for, 101–8; Investigator New Drug approval secured by Scott, 97; as open trials, x, 110, 111–16, 117, 126, 156; Scott's refusal to put limits on, 126
Clostridium botulinum: behavior of, 9–11, 12–14; discovery and identification of, 5, 7–8; durable protective coat of spores, 9–10; ingestion of spores from, 8, 9; longtime presence of, 1production of toxin, 8, 9, 10 (see also botulinum type A toxin); ubiquity of, 9, 12
The Code Breaker (Isaacson), 157
Colby, William, 57, 64–65
Cold War, 58
Collins, Carter, III, 78, 84–85, 95
commercial applications of medical research, 67–68
complications with botulinum toxin treatment, 140, 143, 154
cosmetic applications of botulinum toxin: and Carruthers, 132–37, 140–41; clients returning for, 140; complications with, 140; as driver of market for Botox, 126; facial rejuvenation, 139, 140, 141; FDA approval of, 124–25, 138, 156; indications for, 138; knowledge of facial structure required for, 143; medical applications vs., 121; rules surrounding, 153; and training for cosmetic dermatology, 141–42; wrinkle reduction, 134–35, 138, 141, 142, 145, 156
costs of drug development, x, 128, 129–30
COVID-19, ix
crow's feet, 142

deaths related to botulism poisoning: from blood sausages, 1–2, 3–4, 7; and degree of exposure to toxin, 16; and development of infection, 8, 10–11; epidemic proportions of unexplained, 1–2; from ham, 7–8; incidence of, 30, 147; in infant botulism, 29, 30; Kerner's investigation of, 4; from olives, 21, 23, 24–27, 73; rarity of, in modern times, 29; in Spanish-American War, 20; and understanding of *C. botulinum* in 1943, 44; and Van Ermengem's identification of *C. botulinum* bacteria, 7–8

Delbene family, botulism outbreak in, 26–27

depression, 136, 143

diisopropyl fluorophosphate (DFP), 93–94

Donovan, William, 38, 39, 40

Drachman, Daniel, 82; and botulinum toxin from Schantz, 63, 67; botulinum toxin research of, 5, 68, 90–91, 92; on missed opportunity with patent, 69, 91; recognition owed to, 158; on Schantz's gentle demeanor, 66; Scott referred to Schantz by, 70, 91; and Scott's research, 68–70, 71, 91

drooling (sialorrhea), 149

drooping lids, 142

drug development costs, x, 128, 129–30

Dupixent, 128, 129

Dysport, 96

dystonia: author's work with, 167; blepharospasm (uncontrolled forceful closure of the lids), 112, 120, 121, 142, 143, 144, 149; botulinum toxin indicated for, 149; cervical dystonia, 149, 156; and clinical trials, 112, 115; FDA approval of botulinum toxin for, 121; laryngeal dystonia, 150; limb dystonia, 150; lingual dystonia, 150; and market for Oculinum, 117; oromandibular dystonia, 150; Scott's focus on, 122; treatment of, with botulinum toxin, 133–34

Edison, Thomas, 42

Ehmann, Freda, 27

Eisenhower, Dwight, 43, 51–52

electromyography (EMG), 147

Ellis, Daryel, 111

equine antitoxin, 29, 51

equine encephalomyelitis, Western, 165

Escherichia coli, 7

ethics in medicine and medical research, 59

Evolus, 140

eyes: crossed/misaligned (*see* strabismus); eye muscles, 87–89, *87, 88*; uncontrolled eye movement, 113–14

facial shaping/rejuvenation, cosmetic, 139, 140, 141

facial spasms, 156

FATTOM mnemonic, 13–14

flexion of trunk (camptocormia), 149

"floppy baby" (infant botulism), 8, *12,* 29, 30

Food and Drug Administration (FDA): approval of botulinum toxin, ix, 121–22, 124, 148; approval of cosmetic uses of botulinum toxin, 124–25, 156; and clinical trials, 97, 100–101, 108; and establishment license from, 118; forerunner of, 59; Investigator New Drug (IND) approval secured by Scott, 95–96, 99, 156; predecessor of, 20; restrictions on pediatric patients, 122; and Scott's ongoing research, 100

food safety rules and regulations, 19–22, 29, 44, 59

Ford, Gerald, 50

Ford, John, 39

forehead lines, 142

frown lines, 142

Gahris, Helen Sebring, 24

Galderma, 140

Gatorade, 127

George, Kristi, 152–54

George VI, King of Great Britain, 38

glabellar lines, 142

golf ball chin, 142

Goss, Porter J., 40

Gottlieb, Sidney, 48–49, 50, 51, 52, 53

grinding/clenching of jaw, 139

gummy smile, 142

Guyton, Arthur, *79;* background of, 166; biological weapons research of, 44–45;

and Brooks's research, 67; at Camp Detrick, 69; nerve transmission theory of, 5; recognition owed to, 158; on role of acetylcholine, 70
Guyton, David, 79, 166

handwashing, importance of, 6
Hanke, C. William "Bill," 138–39, 140, 141, 142, 143
Hayden, Sterling, 39
headaches, 139, 143, 150–51
Heinz, 19
Helms, Richard, 57
hemifacial spasms, 142, 149, 152
Hess-Lancaster screen, 161
Hippocratic Oath, 59
Hitler, Adolf, 36–37, 42, 67
Hobart, Garrett, 20
honey, 12
Honeychurch, Dennis, 99, 118
Hooper Foundation, 27
Hoover, J. Edgar, 39, 40
human immune globulin, 29
Humira, 128

Indiana University Medical Center, 138
Indian maharajas, 3
indications for botulinum toxin, 136, 142–43, 144–45, 148–50
infant botulism "floppy baby," 8, 12, 29, 30
inorganic form of botulinum toxin, 160
insurance companies, 152, 153, 154
International Spy Museum, Washington, DC, 53
International Strabismological Association, 111
Investigator New Drug (IND) approval secured by Scott, 95–96, 97, 99, 156
Isaacson, Walter, 157

James Whitcomb Riley Hospital for Children, 112
Jampolsky, Arthur: and Drachman's research, 68; influence on Scott's research, 76, 78, 84–85; and Maumenee's research,

90, 91; and primate studies, 90; and Smith-Kettlewell Eye Research Institute, 83
Jankovic, Joseph, 144, 145, 148
Jean and Alistair Carruthers Award, 141
Jefferson, Thomas, 27
Jeuveau, 96
Johnson, Eric, 56, 63, 66–67, 70, 82
The Jungle (Sinclair), 20–21

Kérner, Justinus, *80, 81*; anticipation of therapeutic uses for toxin, ix, 2, 5, 132, 133, 155, 163; background of, 163; and botulism poisoning outbreak, 3–5, 132; klecksographs of, *81, 164*; poem of, 163–64; recognition owed to, 158; and Scott's research, 133; and understanding of botulism poisoning, 17
Kettlewell, William A., 84
Khrushchev, Nikita, 51–52
Kincaid, John, 152
Kinzer, Stephen, 47, 51
Koch, Robert, 7–8

Lactobacillus, 6
Lamanna, Carl, 5, 44, 158
laryngeal dystonia/laryngeal spasm (spasmodic dysphonia), 145, 150
Lehmer, Jackie, 157, 160, 161
Lehmer, Owen, 161
Leo VI, Emperor of Byzantium, 3
Lillehei, C. Walton, 75
limb dystonia/limb spasticity, 150, 156
Lindbergh, Charles, 37
lingual dystonia, 150
Lumumba, Patrice, 53, 58
lysergic acid (LSD), 47, 49–50

Magoon, Elbert, 86
masseter muscle enlargement, 142
Maumenee, Edward, 68, 90, 91
McCannel, Malcolm A., 110
McKinley, William, 19, 23
meige syndrome, 143
Merck, George W., 42
Merz, 139, 140

rules and regulations around scientific research, 45
rules for food safety, 19–22, 44

salivary (parotid) gland enlargement, 143
Salmonella, 7
Sandoz pharmaceutical company, 49
San Francisco Eye Research Institute, 83
Sanofi/Regeneron, 128
The Saw (Kérner), 163–64
saxitoxin (shellfish toxin): assassination plans involving, 57; at Camp Detrick, 44, 45, 51, 52–53, 57, 61–62; and Church Committee hearings, 61–62; Schantz's maintenance of samples of, 45; and suicide option for U-2 pilots, 52–53
Schantz, Edward, 82; at Camp Detrick research facility, 45; culture perfected and maintained by, 5; as custodian of toxins, 45, 51, 55–56, 59, 60, 61–65, 66; honor system for drug dispersal, 62; personality of, 66–67; recognition owed to, 158; and records on distribution of toxins, 63–64; royalty received by, 121, 129; rules circumvented by, 47; Scott referred by Drachman to, 70, 91; and Scott's research, 45, 56, 63, 65, 67–68, 70–71, 92, 96, 99; Senate hearing testimony of, 51, 54, 58, 60–65; at University of Wisconsin-Madison, 45, 56, 63, 66; wide distribution of botulinum toxin, 125
Scott, Alan Brown: and American Ophthalmologic Society, 106; author's work with, 110–11; and botulinum toxin from Schantz, 45, 56, 63, 65, 67–68, 70–71, 92, 96, 99; and bupivacaine with botulinum toxin, 157; business acumen of, 122, 127, 155; business of (*see* Oculinum); at Camp Detrick research facility, 45; career path of, 1, 75; and Carruthers, 132–33, 141; central role of, in botulinum toxin research, 68–69, 157–58; clinical practice of, 5, 77, 83; clinical trials of (*see* clinical trials); death of, x, 157, 160; and Drachman's research, 68–69, 90–91; education of,

74–76eye alignment treatment sought by, 1 (*see also* strabismus); and eye muscles, 155; and FDA, ix, 100; as first practitioner to use botulinum toxin, 1, 2, 74, 156, 158; first report on research issued by, 93–95; forebears of, 72–73; goals of, 124, 155, 157, 158; house mortgaged for funding, 99, 124, 129; ingenuity and work ethic of, 2, 5, 69, 106; on inorganic form of botulinum toxin, 160; Investigator New Drug (IND) approval secured by, 95–96, 97, 156; and Jankovic, 145; marriage and family of, 75, 161; and nervous system, 121–22; NIH grant proposal of, 2; Oculinum established by, 108, 118, 129, 156; Oculinum sold to Allergan, 45, 63, 108, 124, 125, 127, 157; and patent for work of, 69–70, 118, 125, 156; and pediatric cases, 125–26; personality of, x, 155, 157; primate studies, 56, 92–96, 97, 156; recognition owed to, 158; and Strabismus Research Foundation, 122, 157; Teflon-coated recording needles of, 86, 95, 112, 147; and treatments unrelated to strabismus, 94–95, 109–10, 122, 125, 126, 144–45, 156; trustworthiness of, 86; and wrinkle reduction, 138; youth of, 74
Scott, Helen Elizabeth, 73–74
Scott, Ruth, 75, 76, 77, 95, 99, 161
shellfish toxin. *See* saxitoxin
sialorrhea (drooling), 149
Sinclair, Upton, 20–21
Smith, Clement J., 83–84
Smith-Kettlewell Eye Research Institute: and clinical trials, 98; distribution of toxin discontinued by, 156; and donations to offset costs, 120; downsizing of, 122; and drug development costs, 129–30; establishment of, 83; eye muscle studies performed at, 87–89, *87*, *88*; financial backers of, 83–84; mission of, 84; and NIH grant, 2, 129; and patent for botulinum toxin, 69; primate studies at, 92–96; Scott's work at, 83, 84; as sponsors of Scott's research, 97, 99; and surgery for strabismus, 84–85
somatic nervous system, 146

Van Ermengem, Émile Pierre-Marie, 5, 7–8, 17, 158
Von Noorden, Gunter K., 110

Wangensteen, Owen, 75
weakness caused by botulism poisoning, *10*, 16, 35, *35*, 44
Western equine encephalomyelitis, 165
Wiley, Harvey W., 20
World War II: and biological weapons threat/research, 36, 39–40, 42–47, 68; and Lend-Lease program, 38–39; and Manhattan Project, 42, 46, 49; US's involvement in, 36–40
wounds, open, as source of botulism poisoning, *11*
wrinkle reduction, 134–35, 138, 141, 142, 145, 156
writer's cramp, 150, 152

Xeomin, 96, 139

Eugene M. Helveston, MD, is Emeritus Professor of Ophthalmology at the Indiana University School of Medicine. Dr. Helveston's numerous honors include the Kellogg Scholar Award from the University of Michigan, the Humanitarian of the Year and Silver Recognition Awards from the Indiana Academy of Ophthalmology, and the Outstanding Humanitarian and Life Time Achievement Award from the American Academy of Ophthalmology. He has authored or coauthored three ophthalmology textbooks and over 200 scientific papers and taught and served as a volunteer in fifty countries. In addition, he has written three thrillers and a nonfiction book about youth learning from work. He has two daughters, four grandchildren, and one great grandchild. He lives in Indianapolis.

FOR INDIANA UNIVERSITY PRESS

Lesley Bolton *Project Manager/Editor*
Tony Brewer *Artist and Book Designer*
Brian Carroll *Rights Manager*
Dan Crissman *Trade and Regional Acquisitions Editor*
Samantha Heffner *Marketing and Publicity Manager*
Brenna Hosman *Production Coordinator*
Katie Huggins *Production Manager*
Dan Pyle *Online Publishing Manager*
Leyla Salamova *Book Designer*